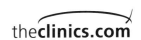

NEUROSURGERY
CLINICS
OF NORTH AMERICA

Interventional Neuroradiology

GUEST EDITORS
Arun Paul Amar, MD
Sean D. Lavine, MD

CONSULTING EDITORS
Andrew T. Parsa, MD, PhD
Paul C. McCormick, MD, MPH

July 2005 • Volume 16 • Number 3

SAUNDERS

An Imprint of Elsevier, Inc.
PHILADELPHIA LONDON TORONTO MONTREAL SYDNEY TOKYO

W.B. SAUNDERS COMPANY
A Division of Elsevier Inc.

Elsevier Inc. • 1600 John F. Kennedy Blvd., Suite 1800 • Philadelphia, Pennsylvania 19103-2899

http://www.theclinics.com

NEUROSURGERY CLINICS OF NORTH AMERICA
July 2005
Editor: Molly Jay

Volume 16, Number 3
ISSN 1042-3680
ISBN 1-4160-2854-4

The ideas and opinions expressed in *Neurosurgery Clinics of North America* do not necessarily reflect those of the Publisher. The Publisher does not assume any responsibility for any injury and/or damage to persons or property arising out of or related to any use of the material contained in this periodical. The reader is advised to check the appropriate medical literature and the product information currently provided by the manufacturer of each drug to be administered to verify the dosage, the method and duration of administration, or contraindications. It is the responsibility of the treating physician or other health care professional, relying on independent experience and knowledge of the patient, to determine drug dosages and the best treatment for the patient. Mention of any product in this issue should not be construed as endorsement by the contributors, editors, or the Publisher of the product or manufacturers' claims.

Neurosurgery Clinics of North America (ISSN 1042-3680) is published quarterly by Elsevier Inc. Corporate and editorial offices: Elsevier Inc., 1600 John F. Kennedy Blvd., Suite 1800, Philadelphia, PA 19103-2899. Accounting and circulation offices: 6277 Sea Harbor Drive, Orlando, FL 32887-4800. Periodicals postage paid at Orlando, FL 32862, and additional mailing offices. Subscription prices are $205.00 per year (US individuals), $315.00 per year (US institutions), $225.00 per year (Canadian individuals), $380.00 per year (Canadian institutions), $265.00 per year (international individuals), $380.00 per year (international institutions), $133.00 per year (US students), and $133.00 per year (international students). International air speed delivery is included in all *Clinics* subscription prices. All prices are subject to change without notice. POSTMASTER: Send address changes to *Neurosurgery Clinics of North America*, W.B. Saunders Company, Periodicals Fulfillment, Orlando, FL 32887-4800. **Customer Service: 1-800-654-2452 (US). From outside of the US, call 1-407-345-4000.** E-mail: hhspcs@harcourt.com.

Neurosurgery Clinics of North America is covered in *Index Medicus*, *EMBASE/Excerpta Medica*, and *Current Contents/Clinical Medicine (CC/CM)*.

Printed in the United States of America.

CONSULTING EDITORS

PAUL C. MCCORMICK, MD, MPH, Professor of Clinical Neurosurgery, Columbia University College of Physicians and Surgeons, New York, New York

ANDREW T. PARSA, MD, PhD, Assistant Professor, Department of Neurological Surgery, Neurospinal Research Center and The Brain Tumor Research Center, University of California San Francisco, San Francisco, California

GUEST EDITORS

ARUN PAUL AMAR, MD, Director of Endovascular Neurosurgery, Yale University School of Medicine, New Haven, Connecticut

SEAN D. LAVINE, MD, Co-Director, Clinical Endovascular Neurosurgery, Columbia Presbyterian Medical Center, New York; Assistant Professor of Neurosurgery and Radiology, College of Physicians and Surgeons of Columbia University, New York, New York

CONTRIBUTORS

FELIPE C. ALBUQUERQUE, MD, Endovascular Neurosurgeon, Barrow Neurological Institute, Phoenix, Arizona

ARUN PAUL AMAR, MD, Director of Endovascular Neurosurgery, Yale University School of Medicine, New Haven, Connecticut

GAVIN WAYNE BRITZ, MD, MPH, Assistant Professor of Neurological Surgery and Radiology, Department of Neurological Surgery and Radiology, Harborview Medical Center, University of Washington, Seattle, Washington

VERONICA L. CHIANG, MD, Assistant Professor, Department of Neurosurgery, Yale University School of Medicine, New Haven, Connecticut

E. SANDER CONNOLLY, JR, MD, Associate Professor, Departments of Neurological Surgery and Neurology, Columbia University Medical Center and New York-Presbyterian Hospital, New York, New York

VIVEK R. DESHMUKH, MD, Endovascular and Cerebrovascular Neurosurgeon, Barrow Neurological Institute, Phoenix, Arizona

LEI FENG, MD, PhD, Clinical Fellow, Department of Radiological Sciences, University of California at Los Angeles, Los Angeles, California

DAVID FIORELLA, MD, PhD, Neuroradiologist, Cleveland Clinic Foundation, Cleveland, Ohio

Y. PIERRE GOBIN, MD, Professor of Radiology, Neurology, and Neurological Surgery; and Director, Division of Interventional Radiology and Neuroradiology, Department of Radiology, New York Presbyterian Hospital, Weill Medical College of Cornell University, New York, New York

BRIAN L. HOH, MD, Resident and Fellow, Endovascular Neurosurgery and Cerebrovascular Surgery, Neurosurgical Service, Massachusetts General Hospital, Harvard Medical School, Boston, Massachusetts

MICHELE H. JOHNSON, MD, Associate Professor, Director, Interventional Neuroradiology, Department of Diagnostic Radiology, Yale University School of Medicine, New Haven, Connecticut

JEFFREY M. KATZ, MD, Fellow, Department of Neurology and Neuroscience, Division of Interventional Neuroradiology, Department of Radiology, New York Presbyterian Hospital, Weill Medical College of Cornell University, New York, New York

DONALD W. LARSEN, MD, Department of Neurological Surgery, Keck School of Medicine, University of Southern California at Los Angeles, Los Angeles, California

SEAN D. LAVINE, MD, Co-Director, Clinical Endovascular Neurosurgery, Columbia Presbyterian Medical Center, New York; Assistant Professor of Neurosurgery and Radiology, College of Physicians and Surgeons of Columbia University, New York, New York

STEPHAN A. MAYER, MD, Associate Professor, Departments of Neurological Surgery and Neurology, Columbia University Medical Center and New York-Presbyterian Hospital, New York, New York

CAMERON G. MCDOUGALL, MR, Director of Endovascular Neurosurgery, Barrow Neurological Institute, Phoenix, Arizona

PHILLIP M. MEYERS, MD, Associate Professor, Department of Neurological Surgery and Radiology, Columbia University Medical Center and New York-Presbyterian Hospital, New York, New York

YUICHI MURAYAMA, MD, Adjunct Assistant Professor, Department of Radiological Sciences, University of California at Los Angeles, Los Angeles, California

CHRISTOPHER S. OGILVY, MD, Director of Cerebrovascular Surgery, Neurosurgical Service, Massachusetts General Hospital, Harvard Medical School, Boston, Massachusetts

DAVID PALISTRANDT, MD, Assistant Professor, Departments of Neurological Surgery and Neurology, Columbia University Medical Center and New York-Presbyterian Hospital, New York, New York

AUGUSTO PARRA, MD, Assistant Professor, Departments of Neurological Surgery and Neurology, Columbia University Medical Center and New York-Presbyterian Hospital, New York, New York

PETER A. RASMUSSEN, MD, Director of Endovascular and Cerebrovascular Neurosurgery, Department of Neurosurgery, Cleveland Clinic Foundation, Cleveland, Ohio

HOWARD A. RIINA, MD, Assistant Professor, Department of Neurological Surgery, Department of Neurology, and Division of Interventional Neuroradiology, Department of Radiology, New York Presbyterian Hospital, Weill Medical College of Cornell University, New York, New York

DOUGLAS A. ROSS, MD, Associate Professor, Department of Surgery, Section of Otolaryngology, Yale University School of Medicine, New Haven, Connecticut

ALAN Z. SEGAL, MD, Assistant Professor of Neurology, Department of Neurology and Neuroscience, New York Presbyterian Hospital, Weill Medical College of Cornell University, New York, New York

GEORGE P. TEITELBAUM, MD, Department of Neurological Surgery, Keck School of Medicine, University of Southern California at Los Angeles, Los Angeles, California

LUCIE THIABOLT, PharmD, Director Strategic Customer and Clinical Programs, Boston Scientific Neurovascular, Freemont, California

FERNANDO VINUELA, MD, Professor and Director of Interventional Neuroradiology, Department of Radiological Sciences, University of California at Los Angeles, Los Angeles, California

CONTENTS

evidence of a healing response in aneurysms treated with Matrix coils. This technology can be further improved through the incorporation of new knowledge on the molecular pathogenesis of aneurysms and the cellular and molecular mechanisms of healing.

Cerebral vasospasm is still one of the leading causes of morbidity and mortality from subarachnoid hemorrhage. Vasospasm refractory to medical management can be treated with endovascular therapies, such as transluminal balloon angioplasty or infusion of intra-arterial vasodilating agents. In our review of clinical series reported in the English language literature, transluminal balloon angioplasty produced clinical improvement in 62% of patients, significantly improved mean transcranial Doppler (TCD) velocities ($P < .05$), significantly improved cerebral blood flow (CBF) in 85% of patients as studied by [133]Xenon techniques and serial single photon emission computerized tomography, and was associated with 5.0% complications and 1.1% vessel rupture. Intra-arterial papaverine therapy produced clinical improvement in 43% of patients but only transiently, requiring multiple treatment sessions (1.7 treatments per patient); significantly improved mean TCD velocities ($P < .01$) but only for less than 48 hours; improved CBF in 60% of patients but only for less than 12 hours; and was associated with increases in intracranial pressure and 9.9% complications. Intra-arterial nicardipine therapy produced clinical improvement in 42% of patients, significantly improved mean TCD velocities ($P < .001$) for 4 days, and was associated with no complications in our small series. We have adopted a treatment protocol at our institution of transluminal balloon angioplasty and intra-arterial nicardipine therapy as the endovascular treatments for medically refractory cerebral vasospasm.

Our understanding of the pharmacology of antiplatelet therapy continues to evolve rapidly. Although the existing data are primarily generated in the setting of interventional and preventative cardiology studies, these data may be extrapolated to guide the rational application of these agents in neuroendovascular procedures. Platelet function testing represents an increasingly available and practical method by which to verify the adequacy of therapy and guide clinical decision making. The optimal application of these agents will undoubtedly improve the risk profile of neuroendovascular procedures, increase the success rate of acute stroke intervention, and facilitate more effective secondary stroke prevention.

The management of interventional neurologic patients in the intensive care unit is based on their underlying disease for the most part. Patients with ischemic stroke are largely managed like patients with ischemic stroke who have not undergone interventional procedures, and the same is true for those with an aneurysmal subarachnoid hemorrhage or intracerebral hemorrhage secondary to an arteriovenous malformation, for example. Having said this, there are some special considerations that require special mention when it comes to managing patients after catheter-based procedures.

FORTHCOMING ISSUES

THE CLINICS ARE NOW AVAILABLE ONLINE!

Access your subscription at
http://www.theclinics.com

ELSEVIER
SAUNDERS

Neurosurg Clin N Am 16 (2005) ix

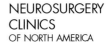

NEUROSURGERY
CLINICS
OF NORTH AMERICA

Preface

Interventional Neuroradiology

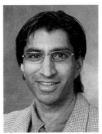 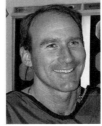

Arun Paul Amar, MD   Sean D. Lavine, MD
Guest Editors

Interventional neuroradiology (INR) procedures are being performed with increasing frequency, both in the angiography suite and in the operating room. These therapies complement and in some cases replace more conventional surgeries of the brain and spine. Although fluoroscopically guided approaches to diseases of the nervous system have existed for decades, their use has grown exponentially in the past several years. Potential reasons for this phenomenon include:

- Recent technical innovations and ongoing device/instrumentation enhancements
- Aggressive marketing campaigns by manufacturers of these devices
- The enfranchisement of neurosurgeons, orthopedic surgeons, and other nonradiologist practitioners
- The growing number of neurosurgeons with hybrid training in INR techniques
- An ever-aging population with commensurate increases in the incidence of diseases best treated by these methods
- The pervasive trend toward therapeutic minimalism

This issue of the *Neurosurgery Clinics of North America* surveys the background, present application, and prospects of several INR procedures. The spectrum of disorders that can be treated with these techniques (ischemic stroke, subarachnoid hemorrhage, vertebral compression fractures, and so forth) is a testimony to the impact of INR therapy and supports its role in the future of neurosurgery.

Arun Paul Amar, MD
Director of Endovascular Neurosurgery
Yale University School of Medicine
333 Cedar Street
New Haven, CT 06520-8082, USA

E-mail address: amar@aya.yale.edu

Sean D. Lavine, MD
Department of Neurological Surgery
Columbia University Medical Center
New York-Presbyterian Hospital
710 West 168th Street, Room 435
New York, NY 10032, USA

1042-3680/05/$ - see front matter © 2005 Elsevier Inc. All rights reserved.
doi:10.1016/j.nec.2005.04.005

neurosurgery.theclinics.com

ELSEVIER
SAUNDERS

NEUROSURGERY
CLINICS
OF NORTH AMERICA

Neurosurg Clin N Am 16 (2005) 463–474

Mechanical Embolectomy

Jeffrey M. Katz, MD[a,b], Y. Pierre Gobin, MD[a,b],
Alan Z. Segal, MD[a], Howard A. Riina, MD[c,*]

[a]Department of Neurology and Neuroscience, New York Presbyterian Hospital,
Weill Medical College of Cornell University, 525 East 68th Street, New York, NY 10021, USA
[b]Division of Interventional Radiology and Neuroradiology, Department of Radiology, New York Presbyterian Hospital,
Weill Medical College of Cornell University, 525 East 68th Street, New York, NY 10021, USA
[c]Department of Neurological Surgery, New York Presbyterian Hospital, Weill Medical College of Cornell University,
525 East 68th Street, New York, NY 10021, USA

Mechanical embolectomy is the latest revolution in the management of acute ischemic stroke (AIS). In 1995, results from the National Institute of Neurological Disorders and Stroke (NINDS) rt-PA Stroke Study Group [1] demonstrated that within 3 hours of AIS onset, carefully selected patients derive significant clinical benefit at 3 months after intravenous administration of tissue plasminogen activator (tPA). Subsequent large placebo-controlled trials, including the European Cooperative Acute Stroke Study (ECASS) I, ECASS II, and ATLANTIS, have unsuccessfully attempted to expand this critical time window from 3 to 6 hours, because the benefit of therapy is outweighed by the risk of intracerebral hemorrhage (ICH) [2–5]. Pooled analysis of the intravenous tPA trials indicates that most of the benefit of intravenous tPA is derived when the drug is administered within 90 minutes of symptom onset, although a favorable outcome based on the 3-month modified Rankin score still persists if the drug is given within 4.5 hours from onset [6]. Stringent inclusion criteria and a restricted time window limit the use of intravenous tPA to only 2% to 6% of stroke patients, however, and only 10% of AIS patients arriving within the 3-hour window are treated with intravenous tPA [7,8].

Patients with large-vessel AIS derive less benefit from intravenous tPA than patients with lacunar or distal embolic strokes, because large-vessel occlusions have less than a 30% recanalization rate with intravenous tPA [9]. The phase IV Prospective Standard Treatment with Alteplase to Reverse Stroke (STARS) study [10] of intravenous tPA use confirmed the findings of others [11] that patients with indicators of large-vessel AIS, including an initial National Institutes of Health Stroke Scale (NIHSS) score greater than 10 and a hyperdense middle cerebral artery (MCA) sign on the baseline CT scan, have less favorable clinical outcomes with intravenous tPA.

Endovascular management of AIS is intended to enhance the degree of large-vessel recanalization and to improve clinical outcome. With cerebral artery occlusion, a central ischemic core undergoes rapid infarction if blood flow is not restored. Surrounding this core is a penumbra of hypoperfused tissue that remains potentially salvageable for several hours. The degree of viability depends on the intrinsic capacity of the tissue to resist ischemia and the extent and duration of regional hypoperfusion. As the time from stroke onset elapses, the amount of viable brain tissue diminishes and the risk of ICH increases. By limiting the amount of drug used, endovascular approaches also aim to lengthen the time window for AIS treatment by minimizing ICH.

Intra-arterial thrombolysis limits ICH through direct thrombolytic infusion by superselective catheterization. The Prolyse in Acute Cerebral Thromboembolism (PROACT) II study demonstrated

* Corresponding author.
 E-mail address: har9005@med.cornell.edu
(H.A. Riina).

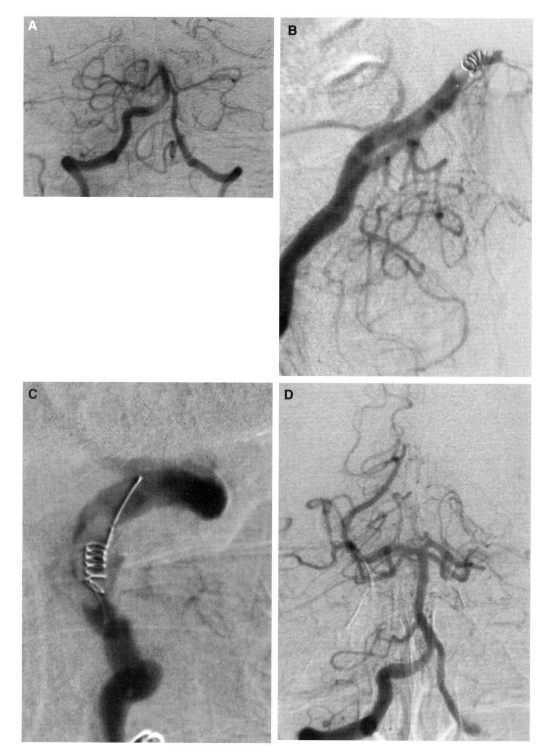

successful MCA recanalization and greater functional independence in patients treated with intra-arterial prourokinase. Clinical benefit was achieved with a number needed to treat of seven at the expense of a 10% symptomatic ICH rate compared with 2% for control patients (and 6.4% in the NINDS intravenous tPA trial) with no mortality benefit [9]. After PROACT II, multiple intra-arterial thrombolysis series using tPA or urokinase have shown positive technical results and clinical outcomes. Based on personal experience and data showing a trend toward lower ICH complications with intra-arterial urokinase compared with intra-arterial tPA [12], we prefer to infuse urokinase intra-arterially. Recent data also indicate the efficacy and relative safety of intra-arterial glycoprotein (GP) IIb/IIIa inhibitors to treat intracerebral artery occlusion refractory to intra-arterial tPA, achieving complete or partial recanalization in 81% of 21 patients treated [13]. Our own experience with intra-arterial infusion of the GP IIb/IIIa inhibitor abciximab has been excellent. Although not approved for clinical use by regulatory agencies, intra-arterial thrombolysis is recommended for carefully chosen patients for the treatment of MCA and basilar artery occlusion by the American Heart Association and American Academy of Chest Physicians [14,15].

Mechanical embolectomy involves the use of novel endovascular devices to physically dissolve and remove thrombus and holds promise for advancing acute stroke management beyond the temporal and population limitations of chemical thrombolysis. Obviating the need for thrombolytic infusion to restore blood flow, mechanical embolectomy is potentially more rapid and aims to broaden the time window for AIS treatment and to expand therapy to patients with contraindications to thrombolysis. This includes patients with bleeding diatheses, recent trauma, surgery, gastrointestinal or genitourinary hemorrhage, noncompressible arterial puncture, ischemic stroke in the prior 6 weeks, past ICH, vascular malformation or brain tumor, and presumed pericarditis or septic embolus.

Mechanical embolectomy has historical precedent. Surgical embolectomy for cerebral artery occlusion was first reported by Welch in 1956 [16]. Multiple cases and small series were reported in subsequent decades that mostly involved embolectomy from the MCA [17–20]. After surgical dissection of the occluded artery, the embolus was located by a bulge and a bluish color of the arterial wall. The artery was occluded proximal and distal to the embolus by temporary clips. An arteriotomy was made through which suction and forceps were used to milk out the embolus. Extracted emboli were described as 1 to 3 cm long and were usually easy to remove with the exception of friable emboli originating from the aortic arch [17,18]. Surgical embolectomy fell out of favor because it was too invasive and required too significant neurosurgical expertise to perform it rapidly enough to support broader appeal.

Devices and techniques

Thrombus retrieval devices

Merci Retriever

In August 2004, the Merci Retriever (Concentric Medical, Mountain View, California) was approved by the United States Food and Drug Administration (FDA) to recanalize cerebral vessels in AIS patients, making it the first clot retriever approved for this indication and the only other treatment that can be offered to AIS patients besides intravenous tPA. The Merci Retriever is a memory-shaped nitinol wire with five helical loops of decreasing diameter at the distal tip that maintains a straight configuration within a microcatheter. Using standard endovascular techniques, a microcatheter is advanced through the circulation to just distal to the occlusive thrombus. The guidewire is then withdrawn and exchanged for the Merci Retriever. As the retriever is directed through the distal end of the microcatheter, preshaped helical loops are released. The retriever is then retracted into the thrombus, ensnaring the clot (Figs. 1 and 2). Once

Fig. 1. (A) A 40-year-old woman presenting with vertigo, dysarthria, dysphagia, and left hemiplegia was found to have a midbasilar occlusion on digital subtraction angiography (anteroposterior view, vertebral injection). (B) The Merci Retriever was used to ensnare the clot 10 hours after symptom onset. (C) The thrombus shadow can be readily seen encircling the Merci device as the clot was retracted through the vertebral artery. (D) After mechanical embolectomy, the basilar artery lumen was restored. Several left posterior cerebral artery branches were still occluded; however, the territory was well perfused by left-sided collaterals and required no further treatment. The patient made a rapid and complete recovery.

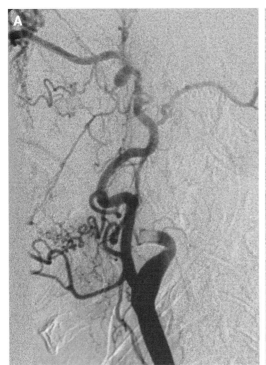

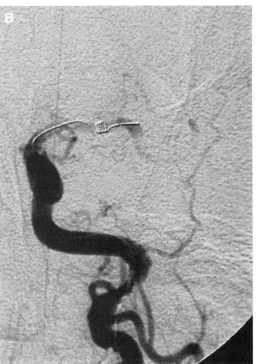

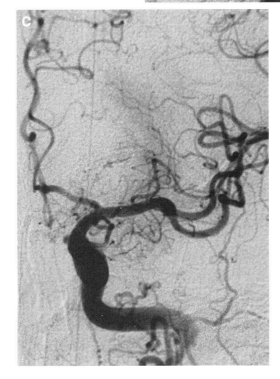

the thrombus is secured, anterograde flow is impeded by inflation of a 9-French balloon guide catheter (BGC). The microcatheter, Merci Retriever, and thrombus are subsequently withdrawn through the BGC lumen and removed from the patient.

In the phase I [21] and II Mechanical Embolus Removal in Cerebral Ischemia (MERCI) Trials [22], 141 patients with a median baseline NIHSS score of 19 (range: 8–40) were treated using the Merci Retriever. Arterial recanalization was achieved in 48% of patients using the device alone, increasing to 57% when the retriever was used in conjunction with intra-arterial thrombolytics. The median procedure time was 1.8 hours. Treated occlusions included those of the MCA in 57%, internal carotid artery (ICA, including ICA "T" [ICA-T] occlusions) in 33%, and basilar artery in 9%. Successful recanalization resulted in functional independence in 47% of patients compared with 10% of those not revascularized and a significant difference in the 30-day NIHSS score (57% versus 15%, a ≥10-point improvement from the baseline NIHSS score).

Neuronet Endovascular Snare

The Neuronet Endovascular Snare (Guidant Corporation, Indianapolis, Indiana) is a nitinol basket attached eccentrically to a microguidewire with more distal than proximal struts that is threaded through a microcatheter past the thrombus [23]. Once the microcatheter is withdrawn, the memory-shaped basket captures the clot and the device is extracted under flow reversal. The device is being investigated in the Neuronet Evaluation in Embolic stroke Disease (NEED) trial in Europe. In a case series of five patients with acute basilar occlusion, two patients were successfully revascularized using the device alone and another patient was recanalized with combined mechanical and chemical thrombolysis [23].

Amplatz Goose Neck Snare

The Amplatz Goose Neck Snare (Microvena Corporation, White Bear Lake, Minnesota), unlike the Merci Retriever and the Neuronet Snare, was designed for endovascular foreign body removal, such as catheter fragments and dislodged aneurysm coils from the cerebral circulation, and not specifically for mechanical thrombolysis in acute stroke. The snare is advanced through a microcatheter and released just proximal to the thrombus, where it assumes a memory-shaped configuration perpendicular to the microcatheter and the vessel. The microcatheter-snare combination is advanced into the clot. The snare is then retracted slightly toward the microcatheter, and the system is pulled back a few centimeters. If the embolus is attached to the snare, as seen by selective angiography, the entire assembly, including the guide catheter, is extracted as a unit under hand suction. Snare size should be equivalent to the diameter of the thrombosed artery. Evidence for the efficacy of the Goose Neck Snare in acute stroke therapy comes from case reports and small series in which the device was used successfully to revascularize patients after failed chemical thrombolysis [24–26] or as a first treatment for large-vessel occlusions [27]. Personal experience with the Goose Neck Snare for the treatment of AIS has been disappointing, however. The snare's loop tends to pull through the arterial clot without adequately engaging the thrombus, making the device insufficient to treat most AIS patients.

Laser thrombolysis

Endovascular Photo Acoustic Recanalization laser system

The Endovascular Photo Acoustic Recanalization (EPAR) laser (Endovasix, San Francisco, California) achieves rapid thrombus dissolution by conversion of photonic energy to acoustic energy at the fiberoptic tip of the device through the generation of microcavitation bubbles [28]. Thrombus emulsification is not a consequence of direct laser-induced clot destruction. The catheter tip is designed with five lateral windows, each with one fiberoptic. Suction of the thrombus is induced by vaporization and reliquification of the cavitation pocket. Once in the catheter tip, the thrombus is emulsified and then ejected out of the catheter into the circulation as microparticles.

Fig. 2. (*A*) A 75-year-old woman presenting with global aphasia and right hemiplegia was found to have a left internal carotid artery (ICA) "T" occlusion with proximal ICA thrombus on digital subtraction angiography (lateral view, left carotid injection). (*B*) The Merci Retriever can be seen in the left MCA surrounded by thrombus (anteroposterior view, left carotid injection). (*C*) After embolectomy, intra-arterial urokinase and abciximab, and petrous carotid angioplasty and stent placement, the ICA, MCA, and anterior cerebral artery were fully recanalized and the patient made an excellent recovery (anteroposterior view, left carotid injection).

The 3-French EPAR microcatheter is guided past the thrombus, the power source is activated, and the laser is drawn back through the thrombus. Continuous infusion of the catheter with indigo carmine, an inert blue dye, is required as a coolant. In a phase I multinational trial [28], 34 patients with a median NIHSS score of 19 were treated. EPAR laser treatment could not be completed in 16 patients (47%) for primarily technical reasons. Sole complete use of the EPAR laser in 18 patients resulted in an immediate recanalization rate of 61% after a mean lasing time of 9.65 minutes. Thirty-day functional independence and a 50% or greater improvement in NIHSS score occurred in 36% of EPAR laser-revascularized patients.

LaTIS neuro laser thrombolysis system

The LaTIS laser device (LaTIS, Coon Rapids, Minnesota) uses photonic energy for thrombus ablation and can be deployed in arteries between 2 and 5 mm in diameter [29]. The optical fiber bundle in the delivery microcatheter uses a pulse dye laser-emitting 577-nm light that is discriminantly absorbed by thrombus and not the vessel wall [30]. An initial safety and feasibility report indicated that the device could not be delivered to the clot in two of the first five treated patients, prompting a revision in catheter design. Rapid clot ablation in one patient after three laser rounds in 49 seconds illustrates the potential utility of this technology; however, a decision has been made not to pursue an efficacy trial of this device [29,30].

Thrombus obliteration devices

Angiojet rheolytic thrombectomy system

The utility of rheolytic thrombolysis has been demonstrated for the recanalization of dural venous sinus thromboses [31–33]. The size and stiffness of the original Angiojet catheter (Possis Medical, Minneapolis, Minnesota) made it inappropriate for intracranial arterial use, although case reports of successful revascularization of basilar and proximal ICA thromboses have been reported [34,35]. The Angiojet uses high-pressure saline jets directed back into the catheter, creating a vacuum that fragments and aspirates the surrounding clot as the device is passed through the thrombus. Although a smaller device was designed to engage the clot in the intracerebral circulation, the phase I Thrombectomy in Middle Cerebral Artery Embolism (TIME) trial has been aborted by the company [29].

X-sizer Catheter System

The X-sizer Catheter System (EndiCor Medical, San Clemente, California) is a dual-lumen catheter containing a helical cutter in its inner lumen that is connected to an external vacuum device. When the system is activated, the helical blades rotating at 2100 rpm fragment the targeted thrombus, which is then suctioned out of the patient through the catheter's outer lumen [36]. The vacuum acts to pull the clot into the catheter tip, thereby averting damage to the vessel wall. The device is currently used during percutaneous coronary interventions and is being modified for thrombectomy in the cerebral circulation.

Percutaneous balloon angioplasty and stenting

Acute angioplasty and stenting is the standard of care for the treatment of acute coronary syndrome (ACS), achieving significantly more rapid vessel recanalization rates and improved clinical outcomes compared with chemical thrombolysis. Angioplasty for the management of AIS has been disappointing, however, mainly because the pathophysiology of AIS and ACS is different. Most ACS result from acute atherosclerotic plaque rupture with subsequent arterial thrombosis. Angioplasty of calcified atherosclerotic plaque results in cracking and dissection of the atherosclerotic lesion, restoring luminal patency that is stabilized by the placement of a stent. In contrast, many AIS arise by embolic occlusion of nondiseased vessels. Angioplasty of fresh embolus tends to displace the clot laterally. When the balloon is deflated, the thrombus rebounds back into an occlusive position. Acute angioplasty and stenting is most successful when treating AIS resulting from hypoperfusion from a stenotic extracranial or intracranial lesion or intracerebral arterial thrombosis from atherosclerotic plaque rupture or when a proximal stenosis precludes advancement of a microcatheter to a distal embolic lesion for intra-arterial chemical or mechanical thrombolysis. Balloon angioplasty is performed by advancing a balloon catheter into the occlusion site, followed by balloon inflation up to 6 atm for 30 seconds. A repeat angiogram is then obtained to evaluate the degree of recanalization. If stenosis and/or occlusion persists, the balloon is inflated successively until complete recanalization is achieved. We prefer to place a balloon-expandable stent after the initial balloon inflation, and then angioplasty the stent until a satisfactory result is obtained (Fig. 3). Several series have shown successful acute intracerebral revascularization using balloon angioplasty alone [37] or in combination with chemical thrombolysis [38] and stenting [13,39].

Ultrasound augmentation of chemical thrombolysis

EKOS small vessel ultrasound infusion system

The EKOS MicroLysUS infusion catheter (EKOS Corporation, Bothel, Washington) is a 2.5-French microcatheter with a distal 2-mm, 2.1-MHz sonographic ring transducer at the tip designed to enhance intra-arterial chemical thrombolysis [40]. A guidewire is passed through the thrombus, and the microcatheter is guided into the proximal portion of the clot using standard technique. Once the guidewire is retracted, the system is activated and thrombolytic is infused through the microcatheter. Ultrasound is transmitted for the first 60 minutes of the infusion. The emitted high-frequency and low-intensity sonographic pulse waves help to modify the thrombus by increasing the surface area for fibrinolysis. Ultrasonic vibration creates local cavitation by producing convection currents and microstreaming at the surface of the thrombus. In the phase I North American Multicenter Safety and Efficacy Trial of the MicroLysUS device [40], 14 AIS patients with a mean NIHSS score of 18 (range: 9–27) were treated. Thrombolysis in myocardial ischemia (TIMI) grade 2 to 3 flow was attained in 57% of patients in the first hour, with a mean revascularization time of 46 minutes. Functional outcome at 3 months included an NIHSS score improvement of 10 points or more and a modified Rankin Scale (mRS) score of 2 or less in 5 of 8 surviving patients.

Ultrasound-enhanced systemic thrombolysis

Despite the loss of 65% to 90% of acoustic energy when 2-MHz ultrasound is transmitted through temporal bone [41], experimental evidence indicates that transcranial Doppler (TCD) ultrasound can enhance intravenous tPA-mediated thrombolysis by increasing drug transport into the clot, diminishing fibrin polymerization, and facilitating tPA binding to fibrin [42,43]. In the phase II CLOTBUST trial [43], 126 AIS patients with a mean NIHSS score of 17 were treated with intravenous tPA and randomized to continuous 2-MHz TCD ultrasound or placebo. Eligible patients had TCD evidence of MCA occlusion. Insonation depths of 35 to 45 mm were used for distal MCA (M2) occlusion, and those of 45 mm or greater were used for proximal MCA (M1)

occlusion. FDA-approved pulsed-wave diagnostic TCD transducers were stabilized over the temporal bone using a standard head frame, and TCD monitoring was instituted for 2 hours. Within 2 hours of tPA administration, 49% of TCD-treated patients had complete recanalization or dramatic clinical recovery (defined as an NIHSS score ≤ 3 or ≥ 10-point improvement) compared with 30% of control patients ($P = 0.03$). Reocclusion was similar in both groups (18% in TCD-treated patients versus 22% in controls). Clinical benefit was abolished at 24 hours; however, a trend toward nondisabled functional outcome (mRS score of 0 or 1) was apparent at 3 months.

Indications and patient selection

Mechanical embolectomy is indicated for AIS patients with significant neurologic deficits who (1) present after 3 hours from symptom onset and thus are not candidates for intravenous tPA, (2) present within 3 hours from symptom onset and have contraindications for systemic tPA, (3) fail to recanalize or to significantly recover clinically after systemic thrombolysis, and (4) have an angiographically demonstrable occlusion of an accessible vessel, including the ICA; M1 or M2 MCA branches; and vertebral, basilar, or posterior cerebral arteries. What constitutes a significant neurologic deficit is debated, because different studies use different minimum NIHSS scores as inclusion criteria. The MERCI investigators [21,22] used an NIHSS score of 10 or greater, and the North American EKOS MicroLysUS trial [40] chose an NIHSS score of 8 or greater as a selection condition. In contrast, a minimum NIHSS score of 4 was chosen by the PROACT II investigators [9] and the phase I study of the EPAR laser system [28]. Additionally, some patients with large-vessel occlusion have minimal, transient or fluctuating symptoms at first presentation as a consequence of adequate collaterals that are maximally autoregulated but then deteriorate clinically as cerebral blood flow fails. Patients with isolated aphasia or neglect attributable to proximal MCA occlusion or stenosis may not qualify for endovascular therapy based on NIHSS criteria; yet, a large area of cerebral tissue may be at risk for infarction if percutaneous intervention is not instituted.

The advantage of noninvasive imaging modalities for selecting optimal patients for endovascular therapy is debated. Theoretically, to obtain maximal clinical benefit of revascularization, patients should have a small infarct core with a large

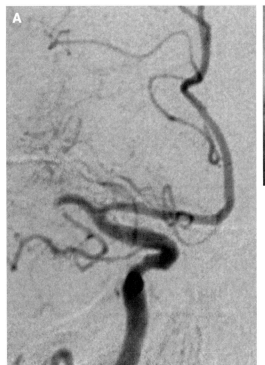

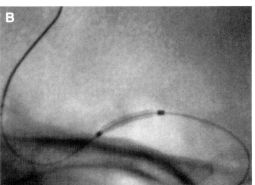

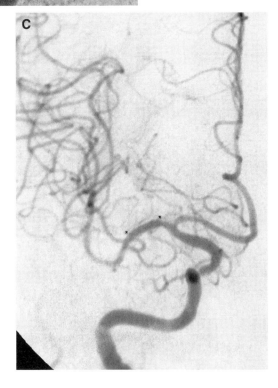

perfusion deficit (penumbra) that would benefit from reperfusion. Two main imaging modalities are currently being investigated and used in clinical practice for this purpose. These have the potential to eliminate the thrombolytic time window and replace it with the tissue window.

MRI acute stroke protocol

Multiparametric MRI stroke protocols combining diffusion-weighted imaging (DWI), perfusion-weighted imaging (PWI), and magnetic resonance angiography (MRA) are useful at identifying tissue at risk [44]. DWI is more sensitive than CT at identifying early infarcted brain tissue (infarct core) [45]. Conflicting data indicate that DWI abnormalities may be reversible in up to 45% of patients after revascularization [46,47]. This reversibility is frequently partial and not permanent and may be dependent on a threshold apparent diffusion coefficient value [47,48]. Combined with vessel occlusion on MRA and PWI qualitative measurement of cerebral blood flow (CBF), a DWI/PWI mismatch can identify tissue at risk and is predictive of which patients are likely to achieve the most benefit from thrombolysis [49] even when intravenous thrombolytic is given up to 9 hours from stroke onset [50]. A DWI/PWI mismatch is evident in nearly 70% of patients imaged within 6 hours from stroke onset [44]. In the absence of a mismatch, patients are less likely to benefit from revascularization. In a retrospective analysis of MERCI penumbra data on 23 patients, the presence of a DWI/PWI mismatch of 20% or greater (14 patients) was associated with clinical benefit from revascularization based on 30-day mRS score (mean mRS score of 1.3 versus 5 in patients with and without a mismatch, respectively) [51]. MR Rescue, a multicenter prospective trial, is currently randomizing patients to endovascular revascularization with the Merci Retriever versus conservative management after stroke protocol MRI. The study intends to determine whether the presence of a DWI/PWI mismatch of 20% or greater is predictive of outcome in patients revascularized using the Merci device. In addition to DWI/PWI mismatch, recent data indicate that a clinical/DWI mismatch is predictive of early neurologic deterioration and infarct growth [52]. At our institution, we tend to prefer the combination of MRA and a clinical/DWI mismatch before mechanical embolectomy if the patient arrives more than 3 hours from AIS onset. The disadvantages of MRI include slow acquisition time, patient contraindications (ie, cardiac pacemaker), the need for patient tolerance (ie, claustrophobia, patient movement, clinical instability), and the lack of widespread availability.

CT acute stroke protocol

CT angiography (CTA) and CT perfusion imaging (CTP) do not have the same restrictions as MRI, require similar postprocessing times, and are universally available. Unlike PWI, CTP offers quantitative measurements of CBF, mean transit time, and cerebral blood volume (CBV) but is limited to only four brain slices and thus can miss zones of infarction. Threshold values for CTP parameters allow excellent assessment of the infarct core and penumbra [53]. CTA and MRA have equal accuracy in detecting vessel occlusion, and CTA source images significantly correlate with abnormalities on DWI [54]. When windowed appropriately, CTA source imaging is a good estimate of CBV and is useful at delineating the extent of tissue infarction. Disadvantages of CT stroke imaging are the need for intravenous contrast and large-bore intravenous access and the limited scope of CTP acquisition.

At our institution, use of MRI- or CT-based stroke imaging depends on the particular characteristics of the case. Regardless of the time window, if a significant infarct/perfusion mismatch is observed, we generally attempt mechanical embolectomy with or without chemical thrombolysis because of the presumed lower risk of reperfusion ICH. Whether or not patients with a well-defined infarct on DWI or CTA source imaging benefit from mechanical embolectomy, even if they arrive within a few hours of stroke onset, is not clear.

Fig. 3. A 69-year-old woman with known right MCA stenosis presented with worsening left hemiparesis and was treated with intravenous heparin and induced hypertension with symptom improvement. Marked hypoperfusion was still found by CT perfusion on hypertensive therapy, however. (A) Digital subtraction angiogram disclosed right MCA occlusion (anteroposterior view, right carotid injection). (B) Balloon angioplasty was performed, followed by stent placement. (C) Intracranial stent deployment maintained a patent MCA (* demarcates stent borders).

Risks of mechanical embolectomy

Reperfusion hemorrhage

The predominant risks of mechanical embolectomy are related to reperfusion injury or to complications of the endovascular device. Extrapolating from intra-arterial thrombolysis studies, the presence and extent of reperfusion hemorrhage after revascularization depends on several factors, including the duration and degree of ischemia; the size and location (ie, basal ganglia involvement) of the infarct core; the pretreatment NIHSS score; and the clinical propensity of the patient for bleeding, including inherent or iatrogenic coagulopathy, uncontrolled hypertension, hyperglycemia, and the existence of previous microhemorrhages on gradient echo MRI [12,55,56]. Whether any of these markers translates into the risk of reperfusion hemorrhage after mechanical embolectomy is not known. Anecdotally, pretreatment use of intravenous tPA or concurrent infusion of intra-arterial thrombolytic or GP IIb/IIIa inhibitors increases the risk of ICH with mechanical embolectomy, although the detrimental contribution of intra-arterial GP IIb/IIIa inhibitor seems to be negligible in most series [13]. In the combined MERCI I and II data, symptomatic ICH occurred in 9% of patients and was most commonly subsequent to ICA/ICA-T revascularization (17%) compared with 6% in MCA procedures and 0% in vertebrobasilar procedures [22]. Limited data on angioplasty and stenting for AIS provide reperfusion hemorrhage rates of 0% to 13% [37–39]. Symptomatic ICH complicated EPAR laser treatment in 6% of 34 patients [28]. There was no difference in the symptomatic ICH rate between TCD- and non-TCD–treated patients in the CLOTBUST study [43]. Mortality consequent to symptomatic reperfusion hemorrhage after endovascular intervention is dismal, reaching 83% in the PROACT II trial [55].

Device-related complications

Complications of mechanical embolectomy devices can be categorized as angiography related or device related. The rate of complications and how effectively they are managed depend on the experience of the operator. Adverse events include failure to deploy the device, device fracture, vessel dissection, arterial perforation, vasospasm, thromboembolism to an uninvolved arterial territory, cardiac arrhythmia (particularly bradycardia), and allergic reaction to contrast dye. Device-related complications occurred in 5.7% of 141 Merci Retriever–treated patients, and half of these represented anterior cerebral artery embolization from MCA revascularization [22]. The EPAR laser could not be deployed successfully in 35% of 34 patients, and 1 patient had a fatal outcome from device-related vessel rupture [28]. The EKOS MicroLysUS catheter was associated with one device failure from a cracked sonography element among 14 AIS treatments [40]. Arterial dissection occurred in 6% and asymptomatic thromboembolism events occurred in 11% of 18 patients treated with intracranial angioplasty [13]. These individual series data indicate that mechanical embolectomy is associated with a low risk of symptomatic device and angiography-related complications and, importantly, that few patients are worse off after endovascular intervention for AIS.

Summary

Mechanical embolectomy devices for AIS are advancing rapidly in design and indications for use. Currently, the Merci Retriever is the only FDA-approved device for clinical use in AIS. In the near future, the endovascular armamentarium should continue to expand as existing embolectomy devices are enhanced, novel devices are developed, and prospective trials to demonstrate efficacy and safety are performed and completed. Additionally, the expanding use of MRI- and CT-based stroke protocols should help to broaden the numbers of patients eligible for AIS intervention and improve patient selection. Hopefully, this will translate into improved clinical and functional outcomes by simultaneously diminishing reperfusion hemorrhage and augmenting the extent of cerebral tissue preservation.

References

[1] The National Institute of Neurological Disorders and Stroke rt-PA Stroke Study Group. Tissue plasminogen activator for acute ischemic stroke. N Engl J Med 1995;333:1581–7.

[2] Hacke W, Kaste M, Fieschi C, et al, for the ECASS Study Group. Intravenous thrombolysis with recombinant tissue plasminogen activator for acute hemispheric stroke: the European Cooperative Acute Stroke Study (ECASS). JAMA 1995;274:1017–25.

[3] Hacke W, Kaste M, Fieschi C, et al. Randomised double-blind placebo-controlled trial of thrombolytic therapy with intravenous alteplase in acute

ischaemic stroke (ECASS II). Lancet 1998;352: 1245–51.

[4] Clark WM, Albers GW, Madden KP, et al. The rt-PA (alteplase) 0- to 6-hour acute stroke trial, part A (A0267g): results of a double-blind, placebo-controlled, multicenter study. Stroke 2000;31:811–6.

[5] Clark WM, Wissman S, Albers GW, et al, for the ATLANTIS Study Investigators. Recombinant tissue-type plasminogen activator (alteplase) for ischemic stroke 3 to 5 hours after symptom onset: the ATLANTIS study—a randomized controlled trial. JAMA 1999;282:2019–26.

[6] ATLANTIS, ECASS, and NINDS rt-PA Study Group Investigators. Association of outcome with early stroke treatment: pooled analysis of ATLANTIS, ECASS, and NINDS rt-PA stroke trials. Lancet 2004;363:768–74.

[7] Katzan IL, Furlan AJ, Lloyd LE, et al. Use of tissue-type plasminogen activator for acute ischemic stroke: the Cleveland area experience. JAMA 2000; 283:1151–8.

[8] Furlan AJ. CVA: reducing the risk of a confused vascular analysis: the Feinberg Lecture. Stroke 2000; 31:1451–6.

[9] Furlan A, Higashida R, Wechsler L, et al. Intra-arterial prourokinase for acute ischemic stroke. The PROACT II study: a randomized controlled trial: prolyse in acute cerebral thromboembolism. JAMA 1999;282:2003–11.

[10] Albers GW, Bates VE, Clark WM, et al. Intravenous tissue-type plasminogen activator for treatment of acute stroke: the Standard Treatment with Alteplase to Reverse Stroke (STARS) study. JAMA 2000;283: 1145–50.

[11] Tomsick T, Brott T, Barsan W, et al. Prognostic value of the hyperdense middle cerebral artery sign and stroke scale score before ultraearly thrombolytic therapy. AJNR Am J Neuroradiol 1996;17(1):79–85.

[12] Kidwell CS, Saver JL, Carneado J, et al. Predictors of hemorrhagic transformation in patients receiving intra-arterial thrombolysis. Stroke 2002;33: 717–24.

[13] Deshmukh VR, Fiorella DJ, Albuquerque FC, et al. Intra-arterial thrombolysis for acute ischemic stroke: preliminary experience with platelet glycoprotein IIb/IIIa inhibitors as adjunctive therapy. Neurosurgery 2005;56(1):46–55.

[14] Adams HP, Adams RJ, Brott T, et al. Guidelines for the early management of patients with ischemic stroke: a scientific statement from the Stroke Council of the American Stroke Association. Stroke 2003; 34:1056–83.

[15] Albers GW, Amarenco P, Easton JD, et al. Antithrombotic and thrombolytic therapy for ischemic stroke: the Seventh ACCP Conference on Antithrombotic and Thrombolytic Therapy. Chest 2004; 126(3 Suppl):483S–512S.

[16] Welch K. Excision of occlusive lesions of the middle cerebral artery. J Neurosurg 1956;13:73–80.

[17] Meyer FB, Piepgras DG, Sundt TJ, et al. Emergency embolectomy for acute occlusion of the middle cerebral artery. J Neurosurg 1985;62:639–47.

[18] Opalak ME, Chehrazi BB, Boggan JE. Emergency intracranial thrombo-endarterectomy for acute middle cerebral artery embolus. Microsurgery 1988; 9(3):188–93.

[19] Kitami K, Tsuchida H, Sohma T, et al. Emergency embolectomy in embolic occlusion of the middle cerebral artery. No Shinkei Geka 1988;16(8):977–82.

[20] Dolenc V, Tivada I, Skaric I, et al. Direct microsurgical intra-arterial procedures on ICA and MCA. Neurosurg Rev 1983;6:7–12.

[21] Gobin YP, Starkman S, Duckwiler GR, et al. MERCI 1: a phase 1 study of mechanical embolus removal in cerebral ischemia. Stroke 2004;35: 2848–54.

[22] Gobin YP, for the MERCI Investigators. Result of the MERCI (Mechanical Embolus Removal in Cerebral Ischemia) Trial [abstract]. Am J Cardiol 2004; 94(6A):128E.

[23] Mayer TE, Hamann GF, Brueckmann HJ. Treatment of basilar artery embolism with a mechanical extraction device: necessity of flow reversal. Stroke 2002;33:2232–5.

[24] Chopko BW, Kerber C, Wong W, et al. Transcatheter snare removal of acute middle cerebral artery thromboembolism: technical case report. Neurosurgery 2000;46:1529–31.

[25] Kerber CW, Barr JD, Berger RM, et al. Snare retrieval of intracranial thrombus in patients with acute stroke. J Vasc Interv Radiol 2002;13:1269–74.

[26] Fourie P, Duncan IC. Microsnare-assisted mechanical removal of intraprocedural distal middle cerebral arterial thromboembolism. AJNR Am J Neuroradiol 2003;24:630–2.

[27] Wikholm G. Transarterial embolectomy in acute stroke. AJNR Am J Neuroradiol 2003;24:892–4.

[28] Berlis A, Lutsep H, Barnwell S, et al. Mechanical thrombolysis in acute ischemic stroke with endovascular photoacoustic recanalization. Stroke 2004;35: 1112–6.

[29] Lutsep HL. Mechanical thrombolysis in acute stroke. eMedicine J 2004; Available at: http://www.emedicine.com. Last updated October 26, 2004. Accessed January 11, 2005.

[30] Clark WM, Buckley LA, Nesbit GM. Intraarterial laser thrombolysis therapy for clinical stroke: a feasibility study [abstract]. Stroke 2000;31:307.

[31] Chow K, Gobin YP, Saver J, et al. Endovascular treatment of dural sinus thrombosis with rheolytic thrombectomy and intra-arterial thrombolysis. Stroke 2000;31:1420–5.

[32] Opatowsky MJ, Morris PP, Regan JD, et al. Rapid thrombectomy of superior sagittal sinus and transverse sinus thrombosis with a rheolytic catheter device. AJNR Am J Neuroradiol 1999;20:414–7.

[33] Dowd CF, Malek AM, Phatouros CC, et al. Application of a rheolytic thrombectomy device in the

treatment of dural sinus thrombosis: a new technique. AJNR Am J Neuroradiol 1999;20:568–70.

[34] Mayer TE, Hamann GF, Brueckmann HJ. Experience with a waterjet thrombectomy device in cerebrovascular disease [abstract]. Presented at the American Society of Neuroradiology 39th Annual Meeting. Boston, April 23–27, 2001.

[35] Bellon RJ, Putman CM, Budzik RF, et al. Rheolytic thrombectomy of the occluded internal carotid artery in the setting of acute ischemic stroke. AJNR Am J Neuroradiol 2001;22:526–30.

[36] Beran G, Lang I, Schreiber W, et al. Intracoronary thrombectomy with the X-Sizer Catheter System improves epicardial flow and accelerates ST-segment resolution in patients with acute coronary syndrome: a prospective, randomized, controlled study. Circulation 2002;105:2355–60.

[37] Nakano S, Yokogami K, Ohta H, et al. Direct percutaneous transluminal angioplasty for acute middle cerebral artery occlusion. AJNR Am J Neuroradiol 1998;19:767–72.

[38] Ringer AJ, Qureshi AI, Fessler RD, et al. Angioplasty of intracranial occlusion resistant to thrombolysis in acute ischemic stroke. Neurosurgery 2001;48:1282–8.

[39] Ramee SR, Subramanian R, Felberg RA, et al. Catheter-based treatment for patients with acute ischemic stroke ineligible for intravenous thrombolysis. Stroke 2004;35:e109–11.

[40] Mahon BR, Nesbit GM, Barnwell SL, et al. North American clinical experience with the EKOS MicroLysUS infusion catheter for the treatment of embolic stroke. AJNR Am J Neuroradiol 2003; 24:534–8.

[41] Grolimund P. Transmission of ultrasound through the temporal bone. In: Aaslid R, editor. Transcranial Doppler sonography. Wien: Springer-Verlag; 1986. p. 10–21.

[42] Behrens S, Spengos K, Daffertshofer M, et al. Transcranial ultrasound-improved thrombolysis: diagnostic vs. therapeutic ultrasound. Ultrasound Med Biol 2001;27:1683–9.

[43] Alexandrov AV, Molina CA, Grotta JC, et al. CLOTBUST Investigators. Ultrasound-enhanced systemic thrombolysis for acute ischemic stroke. N Engl J Med 2004;351:2170–8.

[44] Albers GW. Expanding the window for thrombolytic therapy in acute stroke: the potential role of acute MRI for patient selection. Stroke 1999;30: 2230–7.

[45] Lansberg MG, Albers GW, Beaulieu C, et al. Comparison of diffusion-weighted MRI and CT in acute stroke. Neurology 2000;54:1557–61.

[46] Kidwell CS, Saver JL, Mattiello J, et al. Thrombolytic reversal of acute human cerebral ischemic injury shown by diffusion/perfusion magnetic resonance imaging. Ann Neurol 2000;47:462–9.

[47] Schellinger PD, Fiebach JB, Hacke W. Imaging-based decision making in thrombolytic therapy for ischemic stroke: present status. Stroke 2003;34: 575–83.

[48] Schaefer PW, Hassankhani A, Christopher R, et al. Partial reversal of DWI abnormalities in stroke patients undergoing thrombolysis: evidence of DWI and ADC thresholds. Stroke 2002;33: 357.

[49] Röther J, Schellinger PD, Gass A, et al. Effect of intravenous thrombolysis on MRI parameters and functional outcome in acute stroke <6 hours. Stroke 2002;33:2438–45.

[50] Hacke W, Albers G, Al-Rawi Y, et al. The Desmoteplase in Acute Ischemic Stroke Trial (DIAS): a phase II MRI-based 9-hour window acute stroke thrombolysis trial with intravenous desmoteplase. Stroke 2005;36(1):66–73.

[51] Kidwell CS, Starkman S, Jahan R, et al. Pretreatment MRI penumbral pattern predicts good clinical outcome following mechanical embolectomy [abstract]. Stroke 2004;35:294.

[52] Davalos A, Blanco M, Pedraza S, et al. The clinical-DWI mismatch: a new diagnostic approach to the brain tissue at risk of infarction. Neurology 2004; 62(12):2187–92.

[53] Koenig M, Kraus M, Theek C, et al. Quantitative assessment of the ischemic brain by means of perfusion-related parameters derived from perfusion CT. Stroke 2001;32:431–7.

[54] Schramm P, Schellinger PD, Fiebach JB, et al. Comparison of CT and CT angiography source images with diffusion-weighted imaging in patients with acute stroke within 6 hours after onset. Stroke 2002;33:2426–32.

[55] Kase CS, Furlan AJ, Wechsler LR, et al. Cerebral hemorrhage after intra-arterial thrombolysis for ischemic stroke: the PROACT II trial. Neurology 2001;57(9):1603–10.

[56] Kidwell CS, Saver JL, Villablanca PJ, et al. Magnetic resonance imaging detection of microbleeds before thrombolysis: an emerging application. Stroke 2002;33:95–8.

ELSEVIER
SAUNDERS

Neurosurg Clin N Am 16 (2005) 475–485

NEUROSURGERY
CLINICS
OF NORTH AMERICA

Clipping or Coiling of Cerebral Aneurysms

Gavin Wayne Britz, MD, MPH

*Department of Neurological Surgery and Radiology, Harborview Medical Center, University of Washington,
PO Box 359766, Seattle, WA 98104, USA*

Cerebral aneurysms remain a formidable challenge for neurosurgeons and interventional neuroradiologists. It is estimated that approximately 5% to 15% of all stroke cases are secondary to ruptured saccular aneurysms; therefore, it also remains an important health issue in the United States [1]. Although cerebral aneurysms can present with other symptoms related to their mass effect, such as cranial nerve palsies, their most significant sequela is related to the hemorrhage secondary to their rupture. After this hemorrhage, despite recent improvements in the diagnosis and treatment of cerebral aneurysms, the resultant aneurysmal subarachnoid hemorrhage (SAH) retains a mortality rate of 20% to 40% [2–4]. In those patients who survive, up to 50% are left severely disabled [2–4]. Rehemorrhage is associated with a worse prognosis, with 50% to 85% of patients dying [1,5,6]. The poor outcome is largely related to the effects of the hemorrhage; therefore, the prevention of rehemorrhage in ruptured aneurysms and initial hemorrhage in unruptured aneurysms is the primary strategy for lowering the mortality rate. The goal of preventing the hemorrhage or rehemorrhage can only be achieved by successfully excluding the aneurysm from the circulation.

Two treatment modalities are now available to exclude the aneurysm from the circulation: microsurgical clipping and endovascular coiling. Microsurgical treatment is more invasive and requires a craniotomy, open dissection of the aneurysm, and clipping of the aneurysm. Endovascular coiling is done through a groin puncture, negating the need for a craniotomy, and the aneurysm is excluded from within with microcoils.

The surgical treatment of cerebral aneurysms is the traditional method and remains the "gold standard" in some centers, whereas endovascular coiling is a more recent technique that has been approved by the US Food and Drug Administration (FDA) since the middle of the 1990s. The availability of the two modalities has generated a large amount of controversy and debate with regard to the best treatment of aneurysms. The superiority of either of the treatment options has not been defined, but data are now available with regard to the safety and efficacy of each modality and can be used to decide what is best for individual patients. This decision needs to be made with knowledge of the safety and efficacy data and combined with other important variables, such as the patient's expected longevity, aneurysm factors (eg, size, aneurysm configuration, aneurysm location), and the operator's experience. In addition, it is equally important to consider whether the aneurysm is unruptured or ruptured. This complex decision requires entertaining all the variables, ensuring that patients receive the most appropriate care. This article first addresses the safety and efficacy data and most of the variables that need to be considered and then discusses the management of patients with unruptured and ruptured cerebral aneurysms with respect to clipping or coiling the aneurysm.

Safety of microsurgical clipping versus endovascular coiling

When comparing the safety of the two treatment options, although coiling is not without risk, it seems to be safer than clipping for an individual treatment session. In analyzing the safety data, it is best to evaluate the results of unruptured aneurysms so as to remove the confounding

E-mail address: gbritz@u.washington.edu

associated with the injury related to the SAH. The mortality rate from clipping an unruptured intracranial aneurysm (UIA) is between 1% and 3.8%, and the morbidity rate is between 4% and 12%. A meta-analyses of 733 patients by King and colleagues [7] reported a mortality rate of 1% and a morbidity rate of 4%, and one by Raaymakers and colleagues [8], which included 2460 patients, reported a mortality rate of 2.6% and a morbidity rate of 10.9%, with both decreasing in recent years for anterior circulation aneurysms. The most comprehensive study looking at the risks of surgical treatment was the International Study of Unruptured Intracranial Aneurysms (ISUIA) [9]. In the prospective group of 961 patients who had no history of SAH, the investigators reported a mortality rate of 2.3% at 30 days and 3.8% at 1 year and a morbidity rate of 12% at 1 year [9]. This study also looked at more subtle morbidities, such as neuropsychologic outcomes. Recently, a population-based study evaluating the impact of surgical clipping on survival in unruptured and ruptured cerebral aneurysms reported a 5.5% 30-day and 8.5% 1-year mortality rate in patients with unruptured aneurysms [10]. In addition, those patients who were treated were noted to have a higher than expected death rate compared with the general population, which extended throughout the study period [10].

With respect to coiling, the reported mortality rate after coiling a UIA is between 0.5% and 2% and the morbidity rate is 4% to 5%. A meta-analysis by Brilstra and colleagues [11] that included 1383 patients in 48 studies reported a 3.7% permanent complication rate. Johnston and colleagues [12] compared a cohort of patients with UIAs undergoing surgery and reported a mortality rate of 2.3% versus 0.4% and a morbidity rate of 18.5% versus 10.6%. Johnston and colleagues [13] also reported on 2069 patients treated for UIAs in California between 1990 and 1998 and reported a mortality rate of 3.5% for clipping versus 0.5% for coiling. A recent large meta-analysis of 1379 patients by Lanterna and colleagues reported a mortality rate of 0.6% and a 7% permanent morbidity rate after coiling UIAs [14]. Therefore, the data support the notion that endovascular coiling is safer than microsurgical clipping in patients with a UIA.

The safety of endovascular coiling compared with clipping was further augmented by the results of the International Subarachnoid Aneurysm Trial (ISAT) [15]. This prospective, randomized, controlled trial of neurosurgical clipping versus endovascular coiling in 2143 patients with ruptured intracranial aneurysms demonstrated an absolute risk reduction of 8.7% at 1 year [15]. The results of this trial have generated further controversy [16–18], but it is fair to say that coiling does seem to be safer than microsurgical clipping in ruptured cerebral aneurysms as it is in UIAs.

Efficacy of microsurgical clipping versus endovascular coiling

The appeal of endovascular occlusion of cerebral aneurysms is that it is a less invasive technique and has been shown to be safer than clipping. When managing a patient with a cerebral aneurysm, however, the major goal of treatment in those patients deemed to require treatment is the prevention of hemorrhage or rehemorrhage in unruptured and ruptured aneurysms, respectively, by successfully excluding the aneurysm from the circulation. When comparing endovascular treatment with surgical obliteration of aneurysms, it is believed that the efficacy of endovascular aneurysm occlusion is far less optimal. Aneurysm occlusion using endovascular techniques and surgery is quite different, and this difference may have significant implications for residual aneurysms. In the clipped aneurysm residual, the walls are closely apposed and the remaining aneurysm is completely excluded from the circulation. By contrast, using endovascular techniques, the coils keep the remnant's walls apart. In addition, although experimental models of coiled aneurysms demonstrate that the aneurysm neck becomes entirely occluded by organized thrombus and that the free luminal surface is covered by endothelium, endothelialization is not observed in coiled aneurysms obtained at autopsy or surgery [19]. These various factors mean that any intra-aneurysmal thrombus or coil is exposed to circulating blood, which may allow compaction of the coils or flow around the coil's periphery into the aneurysm sac.

This "efficacy" has been an important factor in favor of microsurgical clipping, because clipping seems to be superior to coiling in achieving those goals over the short and long term. Most series report a 92% to 96% exclusion rate of the aneurysm from the circulation with microsurgical clipping [20–22], as confirmed by postoperative angiography. In addition, this efficacy is sustained with a 0.5% recurrence per year in completely clipped aneurysms [20]. Most importantly, microsurgical clipping also significantly changes the natural history of the disease. In ruptured aneurysms, David and colleagues [20] reported a 0% incidence of rebleeding in 147 aneurysms that were completely clipped over a mean follow-up period of 4.4 years. Twelve (8.2%) of the 147 aneurysms had a residual neck, and they were divided into two groups: dog ear residua and broad-based residua. Patients with the dog ear type had a risk of 1.9% per year of recurrent hemorrhage, and patients with the broad-based type had no recurrent hemorrhage, although they had significant regrowth. Combined, these residuals had a recurrent bleeding rate of 1.5% per year [20] in the 8.2% of aneurysms with residual necks after clipping. The effectiveness of changing the natural history has also been found in UIAs. Tsutsumi and coworkers [23] reported a 0.09% per year hemorrhage risk in a cohort of 114 patients who had completely clipped UIAs.

With respect to endovascular coiling, most series report 40% to 55% complete exclusion, 35.4% to 52% near-complete exclusion, and 3.5% to 8% incomplete exclusion of the aneurysms from the circulation [24,25]. In addition, the long-term durability of endovascular coiling seems significantly concerning, with rates of recanalization reported to range from 20.9% to 28% [25,26]. This recanalization was found to be largely associated with larger aneurysms and those with a poor dome-to-neck (d/n) ratio [25], however. Despite the fact that microsurgical clipping provides a far superior anatomic cure compared with endovascular coiling, coiling has been shown to be effective in changing the natural history of unruptured and ruptured aneurysms. Therefore, complete anatomic cure is not required to change the natural history of a cerebral aneurysm. In the report by Kuether and colleagues [24] on 74 patients with 77 aneurysms that included ruptured and unruptured aneurysms, the authors had no reported hemorrhages over a follow-up period of 1.9 years in those aneurysms that demonstrated complete exclusion. In those with near-complete occlusion, a hemorrhage rate of 1.4% per year was found in the 1.9-year follow-up [24]. The report by Murayama and colleagues [25] on an 11-year experience in 818 patients with 916 aneurysms demonstrated a hemorrhage rate of 1.6% that decreased to 0.5% in the last 5 years. The recent meta-analyses on the treatment of UIAs by Lanterna and colleagues [14] in 1379 patients with an average follow-up time of 0.5 to 3.8 years demonstrated a total of 13 nonprocedural bleeding events occurring in 703 eligible patients. The overall annual bleeding rate was 0.9% per year, and, importantly, only partially occluded UIAs of 10 mm or more bled. Specifically, the bleeding rate of the UIAs larger than 10 mm was 3.5% per year [14]. Therefore, although endovascular treatment does change the natural history of a cerebral aneurysm, it is not superior to clipping and is particularly concerning for larger aneurysms and those that are not completely occluded.

This concern was also demonstrated by a report by Eskridge and Song [27] that evaluated endovascular occlusion in 150 basilar tip aneurysms as part of an FDA multicenter clinical trial that demonstrated a bleeding rate for treated unruptured aneurysms of up to 4.1%. Further addressing the issue of size in the endovascular treatment of aneurysms is a study by Malisch and colleagues [28] that demonstrated a 4% incidence of post–Guglielmi detachable coil embolization hemorrhages in patients with large aneurysms and a 33% incidence in giant aneurysms. Therefore, using current endovascular techniques, although endovascular occlusion is effective, it does seem that it is a less effective mode of therapy than surgical treatment, particularly in large aneurysms and those with an unfavorable d/n ratio.

Patient factors: patient's life expectancy (age, comorbidities, family history, and World Federation of Neurological Societies grade)

It has well been described that advancing age is associated with a worse outcome in ruptured and unruptured aneurysms [9,29]. This was particularly well illustrated in the ISUIA, which demonstrated a combined morbidity and mortality rate of 6.5% for patients less than 45 years old, 14.4% for patients 45 to 65 years old, and 32% for patients greater than 64 years old in those patients undergoing surgical clipping [9]. Similar finding have been reported with endovascular coiling, but the effects seem to be less significant with endovascular coiling in older patients [29,30]. In managing a patient with a cerebral aneurysm, however, age is only one of the factors that need to be considered. This is one area of medicine today that truly requires an individual evaluation when determining care.

This is particularly important in that two modes of therapy are now available, each with its own advantages and disadvantages, that can be used to facilitate appropriate care for the individual patient. For example, it may be more appropriate for an elderly patient or a patient with severe comorbidities with a limited life expectancy to receive no specific treatment or a treatment that is safe than one that provides decades of cure. Similarly, a young patient may forego a safer treatment for one that is more permanent.

Therefore, when evaluating the patient with a cerebral aneurysm, the patient's life expectancy should be estimated. The patient's life expectancy is related to age, associated comorbidities, and family history of illnesses and longevity. Based on these variables, the author divides his patients into those with long, intermediate, and short life expectancies. A long life expectancy would be exemplified by a patient who is expected to live longer than 16 years, an intermediate life expectancy by a patient who is expected to live 5 to 15 years, and a short life expectancy by a patient who is expected to live less than 5 years. The patient's estimated life expectancy is particularly important when dealing with unruptured aneurysms, because the estimated length of life translates into the patient's length of risk from the aneurysm in an untreated (natural history) or treated (no current aneurysm treatment is 100% effective) form.

In patients with ruptured aneurysms, the patient's neurologic condition after the initial hemorrhage is directly associated with survival, and therefore longevity. Multiple grading schemes have been proposed, of which two are the most widely used: the Hunt and Hess scale [31] and the World Federation of Neurological Societies (WFNS) scale [32,33]. Despite this, outcome prediction remains inexact, but these grading scales do provide a guide with regard to survival. WFNS I grade patients are expected to make an excellent recovery; WFNS II and III grade patients are expected to make a good recovery; and in WFNS IV and V grade patients, an unfavorable outcome is expected in greater than 50% of the patients [34]. Therefore, in ruptured aneurysms, in addition to evaluating the premorbid life expectancy, the WFNS or Hunt and Hess grade must be taken into account when deciding on treatment.

Aneurysm factors

Aneurysm size

Aneurysm size is an important factor to consider because it relates to the safety and efficacy of treatment in microsurgical clipping and endovascular coiling. Increased size has unequivocally been shown to have an increased risk with microsurgical treatment [8]. Wirth and colleagues [35]

have demonstrated a linear relation with regard to size and outcome, with a complication rate of 3% for aneurysms less than 5 mm, 7% for 6- to 15-mm aneurysms, and 14% for aneurysms of 16 to 24 mm. Soloman and colleagues [36] showed similar results with microsurgical clipping, with an excellent or good outcome in 100% of aneurysms less than 10 mm, 95% in aneurysms 11 to 25 mm, and 79% in aneurysms greater than 25 mm.

The safety of endovascular treatment is also affected by size on both sides of the size spectrum, with extremely large and extremely small aneurysms having increased complications. Extremely small aneurysms are associated with an increased risk of intraprocedural rupture and a worse outcome. Giant aneurysms usually have a less favorable d/n ratio, are often associated with a higher incidence of a branch vessel origin of the aneurysm neck, and often have intra-aneurysmal thrombus. These factors are associated with parent, branch, or distal vessel occlusion and an associated stroke. Gruber and colleagues [37] demonstrated this and reported a 13.3% procedure-related morbidity rate and a 6.7% procedure-related mortality rate in aneurysms greater than 25 mm with coiling, which is similar to the results with open surgery.

With regard to the efficacy of treatment, surgical clipping is less affected than coiling by increasing size of the aneurysm. Increased aneurysm size is associated with residua, and to a small degree with clipping, and large calcified aneurysms may be treated with parent vessel occlusion with an associated cerebral bypass in select cases with effective results. In contrast, endovascular coiling is associated with significant aneurysm recanalizing and rebleeding with increasing size of the aneurysm [14,37], with rates of postprocedural hemorrhage of 3.5% per year in UIAs larger than 10 mm in size [14].

Aneurysm configuration

Aneurysm configuration is another important factor to consider in the surgical and endovascular treatment of aneurysms. In surgery, the major factors are the size of the neck and the relation of the aneurysm to the major neighboring artery(ies). In patients with wide-necked aneurysms and/or having the aneurysm involve the major neighboring artery(ies), the surgical complexity is increased and experience is required to ensure complete exclusion of the aneurysm with preservation of the parent vessel and its associated branches. With experience, the operator can achieve greater than 90% occlusion of a wide-necked aneurysm safely. Small-necked aneurysms are simple to treat for a neurovascular surgeon.

Aneurysm configuration is even more important in the endovascular treatment of aneurysms, because the occlusion rate of aneurysms by endosaccular packing with coils is influenced by a variety of factors related to the morphologic features of the aneurysm. These include the d/n ratio, size of the neck and dome, shape, and relation to the major neighboring artery(ies). Dense packing of the coils within the aneurysmal sac can be achieved with less risk of migration of the coil into the parent artery when the treated aneurysm has a small dome size, a small neck, and a large d/n ratio, which are conditions that enhance the complete occlusion of the aneurysm with fewer complications [38,39]. In patients with favorable configurations, a high success rate (80%–85%) of complete occlusion can be achieved in such aneurysms [38–40]. In less favorable configurations, the rate of complete occlusion decreases dramatically and is associated with significantly increased complications and decreased efficacy of treatment. The most important factor relating to aneurysm configuration is the d/n ratio, and this is divided into three groups: large, intermediate, and small d/n ratios describing the most favorable to least favorable configuration. Newer techniques have been developed, however, such as stent-assisted coiling, that may change the paradigm of the treatment of wide-necked aneurysms [41,42].

Aneurysm location

In deciding between clipping and coiling an aneurysm, location is of prime importance, because the safety and efficacy of the two treatment modalities are affected by the location of the aneurysm [8,11]. Posterior circulation aneurysms have always been associated with a higher complication rate with microsurgical treatment when compared with anterior circulation aneurysms of similar size [8]. Most published series report mortality that ranges from 3% to 30% and morbidity that ranges from 7% to 40% with surgical clipping [43–46]. In contrast, with endovascular coiling, complications with posterior circulation aneurysms are not significantly different from those with anterior circulation aneurysms [11,47]. More significantly, however, is that complications seem to occur significantly less frequently with coiling

than with clipping in the treatment of posterior circulation aneurysms. Tateshima and coworkers [48] reported procedure-related morbidity and mortality rates of 4.1% and 1.4%, respectively, with endovascular treatment of posterior circulation aneurysms. Eskridge and Song [27] reported on 150 basilar tip aneurysms and had a periprocedural mortality rate of 2.7% and morbidity rates of 5% of ruptured aneurysms and 9% of unruptured aneurysms. Therefore, evidence has shown that endovascular treatment of posterior circulation aneurysms is safer than clipping, and most patients with posterior circulation aneurysms undergo endovascular therapy (Fig. 1). This has been questioned, however, because it has been reported that in expert hands with experience, no increase in risk has been noted in nongiant posterior circulation aneurysms with microsurgical clipping [36].

Unlike posterior circulation aneurysms, middle cerebral artery aneurysms favor surgical treatment. Middle cerebral artery aneurysms often have the aneurysm originating from one or both of the branching vessels and often have an associated unfavorable d/n ratio. This configuration may often result in the aneurysm being unable to be coiled or may allow for migration of the coil into the parent vessel or a branch, resulting in a stroke. Regli and coworkers [49] reported on the endovascular treatment of unruptured middle cerebral artery aneurysms. In that series, 11 (34%) of 34 cases had attempted embolization, 21 (66%) of 34 needed upfront clipping, and 2 (6%) of 34 were successfully embolized, with the remainder undergoing clipping after failed embolization [49]. Therefore, despite major technical advances in imaging and endovascular treatment of cerebral aneurysms, surgical clipping is still the most safe and efficient treatment for most middle cerebral artery aneurysms.

Another location that requires mention is anterior communicating artery aneurysms. These often require dissection around hypothalamic perforators; therefore, with surgical treatment, the question of cognitive dysfunction after treatment has been raised. In a recent study, Chan and colleagues [50] reported impaired verbal memory and executive function with clipping compared with coiling. Finally, in the treatment of paraclinoid aneurysms, microsurgical clipping often requires decompression of the optic nerve to expose the proximal neck; therefore, blindness is always a concern. In contrast to popular belief, however, no difference in complications has been documented in paraclinoid aneurysms, particularly

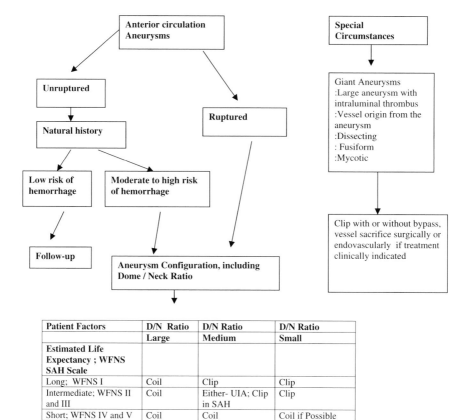

Fig. 1. Algorithm as a guideline in treating anterior circulation aneurysms.

with regard to visual loss with coiling versus clipping [51].

Operator experience

The management of cerebral aneurysms is becoming more specialized, and experience affects outcome, as has been demonstrated in other procedure-related reports in the literature. Unequivocally, improved outcome is found based on the number of cases undertaken and the experience of the surgeon in treating cerebral aneurysms. Solomon and colleagues [52] have demonstrated a 53% decrease in mortality if greater than 10 operations are performed per year. Chyatte and Porterfield [53] demonstrated similar results during the evaluation of outcomes in 449 aneurysm surgical procedures in 366 patients performed by 10 surgeons and found a strong prediction for better functional outcome related to the number of aneurysms treated by

a surgeon. Similar findings have been documented with endovascular coiling of aneurysms [54]; therefore, more and more aneurysms are being treated by neurovascular neurosurgeons and interventional neuroradiologists with an interest in cerebral aneurysms.

Management of unruptured aneurysms

SAH after rupture of a cerebral aneurysm is a devastating condition. In UIAs, prevention of this rupture by surgical or endovascular treatment is believed to be the most effective strategy for lowering the morbidity and mortality rates (see Fig. 1; Fig. 2). All current treatments carry some risks; therefore, in formulating recommendations for treatment of a patient with a UIA, multiple factors have to be considered. The first and probably the most important decision is to evaluate if the patient should be treated at all, because treatment-related complications usually occur at

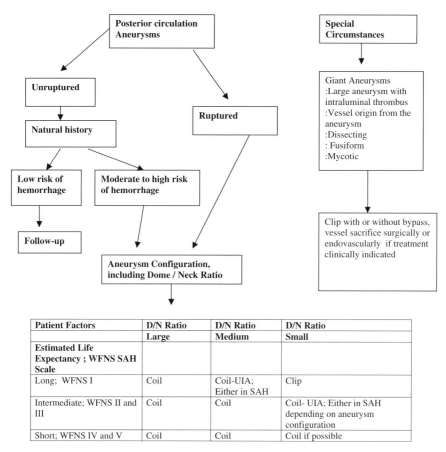

Fig. 2. Algorithm as a guideline in treating posterior circulation aneurysms.

Patient Factors	D/N Ratio	D/N Ratio	D/N Ratio
	Large	Medium	Small
Estimated Life Expectancy ; WFNS SAH Scale			
Long; WFNS I	Coil	Coil-UIA; Either in SAH	Clip
Intermediate; WFNS II and III	Coil	Coil	Coil- UIA; Either in SAH depending on aneurysm configuration
Short; WFNS IV and V	Coil	Coil	Coil if possible

or around the time of the procedure. The indication to treat a UIA is if the risk of the aneurysm outweighs the risk of the treatment. The risk that the aneurysm poses is the natural history of a UIA. Although understanding the natural history of UIAs is critical in the management of patients with a UIA, it is poorly understood, and the risk of rupture has been estimated to be between 1% and 2% per year in multiple studies for aneurysms of average size [55–59]. This continued debate has recently been highlighted by the landmark report from the ISUIA [9], which has suggested a yearly rate of hemorrhage of 0.05%, and recent articles by Asari and Ohmoto [60], Juvela and coworkers [61], Tsutsumi and colleagues [21], and Winn and coworkers [62], which have supported the earlier yearly rate of 1% to 2%.

In treating UIAs, the author divides the risk of hemorrhage into low, moderate, and high risk. Low risk is an estimated natural history of 0.05%

per year or less, moderate risk is an estimated natural history of 0.06% to 2% per year, and high risk is an estimated natural history of greater than 2% per year. Therefore, in those patients with a single UIA less than 5 mm in size, most surgeons do not treat the aneurysm, and the author places those aneurysms in the low-risk category and observes for growth of the aneurysm. An exception to this generalization is that patients with multiple aneurysms, posterior circulation aneurysms, a history of a prior SAH, or a strong family history may have an increased risk of hemorrhage, and the surgeon may consider treating an aneurysm of 4 to 5 mm in size in those situations. Aneurysms ranging from 6 to 24 mm in size are placed in a moderate risk of hemorrhage category. Aneurysms that are larger in size, such as giant aneurysms (>25 mm), have a particularly grave prognosis with a rupture rate of 6% in the first year and 45% within 7.5 years and are placed in the high-risk hemorrhage category [58]. Patients who have a moderate to high risk of hemorrhage should always be considered candidates for treatment.

In those patients who are deemed candidates for treatment, the aneurysm configuration and, in particular, the d/n ratio should be evaluated next. Because almost all intracranial aneurysms can be treated surgically, the plausibility and effectiveness of the endovascular option should be addressed, and the aneurysm configuration provides these data as described previously. Patients are then grouped into those with a large, intermediate, and small d/n ratio describing the most favorable to least favorable configuration, respectively.

All this information is taken into consideration after evaluating the patient's estimated life expectancy. Patients are considered to have a long, intermediate, or short life expectancy. As described earlier, the only time to treat an aneurysm is if risk of rupture over the patient's expected lifespan is greater than the risk of treatment. For example, an elderly and frail patient may not warrant treatment at all even if the patient has a moderate to high risk of hemorrhage, because the risk of the procedure would be higher in an old patient and the length of risk from the aneurysm may be short. In those patients in whom the risk of the aneurysm is worse than the treatment, a treatment option should be discussed with the patient. In those patients, the aneurysm configuration and the patient's estimated life expectancy are calculated with knowledge of the advantages and disadvantages of the two different treatment modalities. As discussed earlier, the advantage of clipping is that it is a relatively safe procedure that is effective in changing the natural history of a UIA in the short and long term. The disadvantage of clipping is that the risk of treatment is higher than that of coiling. The advantage of coiling is that it is less invasive and safer than clipping, but the major limitation is its lack of durability in changing the natural history compared with clipping in those aneurysms that have a less than ideal configuration and in large aneurysms.

Therefore, in anterior circulation aneurysms in patients with a large d/n ratio, endovascular coiling should always be considered as the first line of treatment in those patients with long, intermediate, and short estimated life expectancies, because this treatment provides the patient with relatively effective treatment that is safer than clipping. Some authors may argue that those patients with an estimated long life expectancy should undergo clipping because it has been proven to more durable than coiling. This is a reasonable option for the experienced neurovascular surgeon and the patient. At the other extreme, patients with a long estimated life expectancy or small d/n ratio should undergo clipping, except those patients who have an extremely short life expectancy and in whom coiling is possible based on aneurysm configuration. In patients with a medium d/n ratio and a long estimated life expectancy, clipping would be most appropriate to provide a more durable treatment. In patients with an intermediate lifetime risk, either treatment would be appropriate, and in patients with a short estimated lifetime risk, coiling would be more appropriate.

With regard to posterior circulation aneurysms, in the hands of most surgeons, a higher complication rate is associated with microsurgical treatment when compared with anterior circulation aneurysms of a similar size and is higher than with endovascular coiling. Therefore, in those patients with large and medium d/n ratios, the patient should undergo endovascular coiling regardless of the estimated life expectancy, because endovascular coiling provides a safer treatment that is relatively effective. In those patients with a small or unfavorable d/n ratio, coiling should still be considered in those individuals with a short or intermediate estimated life expectancy because it is still probably safer than microsurgical clipping. In some posterior circulation aneurysms with less favorable configurations, where the aneurysm sac involves one of the posterior cerebral branches, clipping may be the only alternative. Microsurgical clipping should also be performed in those patients with an unfavorable or small d/n ratio with a long estimated life expectancy by an experienced neurovascular neurosurgeon so as to provide the patient with reasonably safe and effective long-term treatment.

Management of ruptured cerebral aneurysms

In ruptured aneurysms, the primary cause of death or disability is related to the effect of the initial hemorrhage, subsequent rebleeding, and associated complications of hemorrhage, such as vasospasm and hydrocephalus. Therefore, in addressing the treatment of a ruptured aneurysm, preventing rebleeding is crucial to prevent further injury to an already compromised brain. Rehemorrhage is associated with an even worse prognosis, with 50% to 85% of patients dying [1,5,6].

The natural history data on ruptured aneurysms suggest that between 20% and 30% of these ruptured aneurysms may rebleed within 30 days [5]. This rebleeding is greatest on day 1 (4%) and then occurs at a constant rate of 1% to 2% per day over the next 4 weeks [63]. After the 4-week period, the rebleeding rate settles down to approximately 3% per year, which is higher than for unruptured aneurysms of a similar size [5]. Therefore, in treating patients with ruptured aneurysms, the primary goal is early, complete, permanent, and safe aneurysm occlusion unless other factors, such as brain death, poor premorbid medical condition, or poor clinical grade, deem this inappropriate.

In those patients who are deemed candidates for treatment, as with UIA, the aneurysm configuration and, in particular, the d/n ratio should be evaluated next. Again, patients are then placed into large, intermediate, and small d/n ratio categories describing the most favorable to least favorable configuration for endovascular therapy. In ruptured aneurysms, in addition to evaluating the patient's life expectancy based on the premorbid status, the patient's clinical condition after the hemorrhage must be considered because this is directly associated with early survival, and therefore longevity. The author arbitrarily places patients into three groups: those expected to survive with no or minimal deficits (WFNS I), those expected to survive with mild to moderate deficits (WFNS II and III), and those possibly not surviving and most likely to have deficits (WFNS IV and V).

As discussed earlier, although endovascular coiling is effective in changing the natural history of ruptured aneurysms, it does seem to be less effective than surgical treatment, particularly in large aneurysms and those with an unfavorable n/d ratio. In ruptured aneurysms, the effectiveness of treatment is particularly vital, because rebleeding is associated with a worse prognosis. Therefore, in treating a patient with a ruptured aneurysm in the anterior circulation, clipping is advocated in those patients with medium or small d/n ratios, except in those patients with a short life expectancy and/or a poor clinical grade after the initial hemorrhage. Endovascular coiling is reserved for those patients with a large d/n ratio in whom complete occlusion can be obtained. In posterior circulation aneurysms, coiling is still the first choice; microsurgical treatment is advocated for those patients with an unfavorable d/n ratio, a long life expectancy, and a good clinical grade and is an option in those with a medium d/n ratio.

Special circumstances

Although most aneurysms can be treated with standard microsurgical clipping or endovascular therapy, some aneurysms require special mention. Giant calcified aneurysms, large aneurysms with intraluminal thrombus, aneurysms in which the vessel is originating from the aneurysm, dissecting aneurysms, and fusiform and mycotic aneurysms need to be evaluated differently. These aneurysms require clipping with or without bypass or vessel sacrifice surgically or endovascularly if treatment is clinically indicated.

Summary

The management of a patient with a cerebral aneurysm is complex, and two accepted treatment modalities are now available. The superiority of either of the treatment options has not been defined, but data are now available with regard to the safety and efficacy of each modality and can be used to decide what is best for individual patients when combined with other important variables, such as the patient's expected longevity, specific aneurysm factors (eg, size, d/n ratio, location), and operator's experience. This complex decision entertaining all the variables should ensure that patients receive the most appropriate care. New developments in the endovascular management of cerebral aneurysms are likely to alter this algorithm.

References

[1] Bederson JB, Awad IA, et al. Recommendations for the management of patients with unruptured intracranial aneurysms: a statement for healthcare professionals from the Stroke Council of the American Heart Association. Stroke 2000;31(11): 2742–50.

[2] Kissela BM, Sauerbeck L, et al. Subarachnoid hemorrhage: a preventable disease with a heritable component. Stroke 2002;33(5):1321–6.

[3] Longstreth WT Jr, Nelson LM, et al. Clinical course of spontaneous subarachnoid hemorrhage: a population-based study in King County, Washington. Neurology 1993;43(4):712–8.

[4] Ruigrok YM, Buskens E, et al. Attributable risk of common and rare determinants of subarachnoid hemorrhage. Stroke 2001;32(5):1173–5.

[5] Winn HR, Richardson AE, et al. The long-term prognosis in untreated cerebral aneurysms: I. The incidence of late hemorrhage in cerebral aneurysm: a 10-year evaluation of 364 patients. Ann Neurol 1977;1(4):358–70.

[6] Nishioka H, Torner JC, et al. Cooperative study of intracranial aneurysms and subarachnoid hemorrhage: a long-term prognostic study. III. Subarachnoid hemorrhage of undetermined etiology. Arch Neurol 1984;41(11):1147–51.

[7] King JT Jr, Berlin JA, et al. Morbidity and mortality from elective surgery for asymptomatic, unruptured, intracranial aneurysms: a meta-analysis. J Neurosurg 1994;81(6):837–42.

[8] Raaymakers TW, Rinkel GJ, et al. Mortality and morbidity of surgery for unruptured intracranial aneurysms: a meta-analysis. Stroke 1998;29(8):1531–8.

[9] Investigators I. Unruptured intracranial aneurysms—risk of rupture and risks of surgical intervention. N Engl J Med 1998;339:1725–33.

[10] Britz GW, Salem L, et al. Impact of surgical clipping on survival in unruptured and ruptured cerebral aneurysms: a population-based study. Stroke 2004;35(6):1399–403.

[11] Brilstra EH, Rinkel GJ, et al. Treatment of intracranial aneurysms by embolization with coils: a systematic review. Stroke 1999;30(2):470–6.

[12] Johnston SC, Dudley RA, et al. Surgical and endovascular treatment of unruptured cerebral aneurysms at university hospitals. Neurology 1999;52(9):1799–805.

[13] Johnston SC, Zhao S, et al. Treatment of unruptured cerebral aneurysms in California. Stroke 2001;32(3):597–605.

[14] Lanterna LA, Tredici G, et al. Treatment of unruptured cerebral aneurysms by embolization with Guglielmi detachable coils: case-fatality, morbidity, and effectiveness in preventing bleeding—a systematic review of the literature. Neurosurgery 2004;55(4):767–75 [discussion: 775–8].

[15] Molyneux A, Kerr R, et al. International Subarachnoid Aneurysm Trial (ISAT) of neurosurgical clipping versus endovascular coiling in 2143 patients with ruptured intracranial aneurysms: a randomised trial. Lancet 2002;360(9342):1267–74.

[16] Britz GW, Newell DW, et al. The ISAT trial. Lancet 2003;361(9355):431–2 [author reply: 432].

[17] Nichols DA, Brown RD Jr, et al. Coils or clips in subarachnoid haemorrhage? Lancet 2002;360(9342):1262–3.

[18] Mohr JP. The ISAT trial. Lancet 2003;361(9355):431 [author reply: 432].

[19] Mizoi K, Yoshimoto T, et al. A pitfall in the surgery of a recurrent aneurysm after coil embolization and its histological observation: technical case report. Neurosurgery 1996;39(1):165–8 [discussion: 168–9].

[20] David CA, Vishteh AG, et al. Late angiographic follow-up review of surgically treated aneurysms. J Neurosurg 1999;91(3):396–401.

[21] Le Roux PD, Elliott JP, et al. Risks and benefits of diagnostic angiography after aneurysm surgery: a retrospective analysis of 597 studies. Neurosurgery 1998;42(6):1248–54 [discussion: 1254–5].

[22] Payner TD, Horner TG, et al. Role of intraoperative angiography in the surgical treatment of cerebral aneurysms. J Neurosurg 1998;88(3):441–8.

[23] Tsutsumi K, Ueki K, et al. Risk of subarachnoid hemorrhage after surgical treatment of unruptured cerebral aneurysms. Stroke 1999;30(6):1181–4.

[24] Kuether TA, Nesbit GM, et al. Clinical and angiographic outcomes, with treatment data, for patients with cerebral aneurysms treated with Guglielmi detachable coils: a single-center experience. Neurosurgery 1998;43(5):1016–25.

[25] Murayama Y, Nien YL, et al. Guglielmi detachable coil embolization of cerebral aneurysms: 11 years' experience. J Neurosurg 2003;98(5):959–66.

[26] Thornton J, Debrun GM, et al. Follow-up angiography of intracranial aneurysms treated with endovascular placement of Guglielmi detachable coils. Neurosurgery 2002;50(2):239–49 [discussion: 249–50].

[27] Eskridge JM, Song JK. Endovascular embolization of 150 basilar tip aneurysms with Guglielmi detachable coils: results of the Food and Drug Administration multicenter clinical trial. J Neurosurg 1998;89(1):81–6.

[28] Malisch TW, Guglielmi G, et al. Intracranial aneurysms treated with the Guglielmi detachable coil: midterm clinical results in a consecutive series of 100 patients. J Neurosurg 1997;87(2):176–83.

[29] Barker FG II, Amin-Hanjani S, et al. Age-dependent differences in short-term outcome after surgical or endovascular treatment of unruptured intracranial aneurysms in the United States, 1996–2000. Neurosurgery 2004;54(1):18–28 [discussion: 28–30].

[30] Birchall D, Khangure M, et al. Endovascular management of acute subarachnoid haemorrhage in the elderly. Br J Neurosurg 2001;15(1):35–8.

[31] Hunt WE, Hess RM. Surgical risk as related to time of intervention in the repair of intracranial aneurysms. J Neurosurg 1968;28(1):14–20.

[32] Drake CG, Hunt WE, Sano K, et al. Report of World Federation of Neurological Surgeons Committee on a universal subarachnoid hemorrhage grading scale. J Neurosurg 1988;68:985–6.

[33] van Gijn J, Bromberg JE, et al. Definition of initial grading, specific events, and overall outcome in patients with aneurysmal subarachnoid hemorrhage. A survey. Stroke 1994;25(8):1623–7.

[34] Rosen DS, Macdonald RL. Grading of subarachnoid hemorrhage: modification of the world World Federation of Neurosurgical Societies scale on the basis of data for a large series of patients. Neurosurgery 2004;54(3):566–75 [discussion: 575–6].

[35] Wirth FP, Laws ER Jr, et al. Surgical treatment of incidental intracranial aneurysms. Neurosurgery 1983;12(5):507–11.

[36] Solomon RA, Fink ME, et al. Surgical management of unruptured intracranial aneurysms. J Neurosurg 1994;80(3):440–6.

[37] Gruber A, Killer M, et al. Clinical and angiographic results of endosaccular coiling treatment of giant and very large intracranial aneurysms: a 7-year, single-center experience. Neurosurgery 1999;45(4): 793–803 [discussion: 803–4].

[38] Debrun GM, Aletich VA, et al. Selection of cerebral aneurysms for treatment using Guglielmi detachable coils: the preliminary University of Illinois at Chicago experience. Neurosurgery 1998;43(6):1281–95 [discussion: 1296–7].

[39] Moret J, Cognard C, et al. Reconstruction technic in the treatment of wide-neck intracranial aneurysms. Long-term angiographic and clinical results. Apropos of 56 cases. J Neuroradiol 1997;24(1):30–44.

[40] Kiyosue H, Tanoue S, et al. Anatomic features predictive of complete aneurysm occlusion can be determined with three-dimensional digital subtraction angiography. AJNR Am J Neuroradiol 2002;23(7): 1206–13.

[41] Benitez RP, Silva MT, et al. Endovascular occlusion of wide-necked aneurysms with a new intracranial microstent (Neuroform) and detachable coils. Neurosurgery 2004;54(6):1359–67 [discussion: 1368].

[42] Chow MM, Woo HH, et al. A novel endovascular treatment of a wide-necked basilar apex aneurysm by using a Y-configuration, double-stent technique. Am J Neuroradiol 2004;25(3):509–12.

[43] Drake CG. Further experience with surgical treatment of aneurysm of the basilar artery. J Neurosurg 1968;29(4):372–92.

[44] Sugita K, Kobayashi S, et al. Microneurosurgery for aneurysms of the basilar artery. J Neurosurg 1979; 51(5):615–20.

[45] Samson D, Batjer HH, et al. Current results of the surgical management of aneurysms of the basilar apex. Neurosurgery 1999;44(4):697–702 [discussion: 702–4].

[46] Morcos J. Distal basilar artery aneurysms: surgical techniques. Philadelphia: Lippincott-Raven; 1997.

[47] Lusseveld E, Brilstra EH, et al. Endovascular coiling versus neurosurgical clipping in patients with a ruptured basilar tip aneurysm. J Neurol Neurosurg Psychiatry 2002;73(5):591–3.

[48] Tateshima S, Murayama Y, et al. Endovascular treatment of basilar tip aneurysms using Guglielmi detachable coils: anatomic and clinical outcomes in 73 patients from a single institution. Neurosurgery 2000;47(6):1332–9 [discussion: 1339–42].

[49] Regli L, Uske A, et al. Endovascular coil placement compared with surgical clipping for the treatment of unruptured middle cerebral artery aneurysms: a consecutive series. J Neurosurg 1999;90(6):1025–30.

[50] Chan A, Ho S, et al. Neuropsychological sequelae of patients treated with microsurgical clipping or endovascular embolization for anterior communicating artery aneurysm. Eur Neurol 2002;47(1): 37–44.

[51] Hoh BL, Carter BS, et al. Results after surgical and endovascular treatment of paraclinoid aneurysms by a combined neurovascular team. Neurosurgery 2001;48(1):78–89 [discussion: 89–90].

[52] Solomon RA, Mayer SA, et al. Relationship between the volume of craniotomies for cerebral aneurysm performed at New York state hospitals and in-hospital mortality. Stroke 1996;27(1):13–7.

[53] Chyatte D, Porterfield R. Functional outcome after repair of unruptured intracranial aneurysms. J Neurosurg 2001;94(3):417–21.

[54] Singh V, Gress DR, et al. The learning curve for coil embolization of unruptured intracranial aneurysms. AJNR Am J Neuroradiol 2002;23(5): 768–71.

[55] Heiskanen O. Risk of bleeding from unruptured aneurysm in cases with multiple intracranial aneurysms. J Neurosurg 1981;55(4):524–6.

[56] Juvela S, Porras M, et al. Natural history of unruptured intracranial aneurysms: a long-term follow-up study. J Neurosurg 1993;79(2):174–82.

[57] Wiebers DO, Whisnant JP, et al. The natural history of unruptured intracranial aneurysms. N Engl J Med 1981;304(12):696–8.

[58] Jane JA, Kassell NF, et al. The natural history of aneurysms and arteriovenous malformations. J Neurosurg 1985;62(3):321–3.

[59] Yasui N, Suzuki A, et al. Long-term follow-up study of unruptured intracranial aneurysms. Neurosurgery 1997;40(6):1155–9 [discussion: 1159–60].

[60] Asari S, Ohmoto T. Natural history and risk factors of unruptured cerebral aneurysms. Clin Neurol Neurosurg 1993;95(3):205–14.

[61] Juvela S, Porras M, et al. Natural history of unruptured intracranial aneurysms: probability of and risk factors for aneurysm rupture. J Neurosurg 2000; 93(3):379–87.

[62] Winn HR, Jane Sr JA, et al. Prevalence of asymptomatic incidental aneurysms: review of 4568 arteriograms. J Neurosurg 2002;96(1):43–9.

[63] Kassell NF, Torner JC. Aneurysmal rebleeding: a preliminary report from the Cooperative Aneurysm Study. Neurosurgery 1983;13(5):479–81.

ELSEVIER
SAUNDERS

Neurosurg Clin N Am 16 (2005) 487–499

NEUROSURGERY
CLINICS
OF NORTH AMERICA

Healing of Intracranial Aneurysms with Bioactive Coils

Lei Feng, MD, PhD*, Fernando Vinuela, MD, Yuichi Murayama, MD

*Department of Radiological Sciences, University of California at Los Angeles,
10833 Le Conte Avenue, Los Angeles, CA 90095–1721, USA*

The birth of Guglielmi detachable coils (GDCs) a decade ago [1,2] has injected new life into the treatment of cerebral aneurysms, gradually changing the management of subarachnoid hemorrhage. More and more medical centers have adopted coil embolization as the first treatment of choice for ruptured aneurysms, particularly after the International Subarachnoid Aneurysm Trial (ISAT) demonstrated the superior safety of endovascular treatment over surgical clipping in patients with ruptured intracranial aneurysms that can be treated with either technique [3]. As this technology goes through its puberty, a shortcoming has become evident, undermining our confidence in its long-term efficacy: large clinical series have shown a high recanalization rate of embolized aneurysms. In 11 years' experience of treating 916 aneurysms at the University of California at Los Angeles (UCLA) [4], the overall recanalization rate is 20.9%. Other groups have reported recanalization rates between 14.7% and 30% [5–7], consistent with the UCLA experience. Large and giant aneurysms are at higher risk of recanalization than small aneurysms. Aneurysms with a wide neck are also more likely to recanalize than small-neck aneurysms. Because the long term follow-up data are still sparse, we do not know the clinical implications of recanalization. Most of the delayed ruptures have been observed in large or giant aneurysms, which are frequently incompletely treated and suffer coil compaction, suggesting that improved obliteration of the aneurysm neck and prevention of coil compaction may be required to treat patients with aneurysms in a definitive manner.

Bioactive (Matrix; Boston Scientific Inc., Fumont, California) coils mark the maturation of this technology from mechanical occlusion to biologic healing of aneurysms. Although the refining of GDC technology produced softer, smaller, and stretch-resistant coils, which allow easier and tighter packing of the aneurysms, no more than 30% of the aneurysm lumen is packed by the coil mass. The rest of the aneurysm lumen is filled with thrombus, which undergoes biologic changes over the first 2 to 3 weeks after treatment to become organized thrombus or fibrous scar. This biologic process thus plays an important role in eliminating the aneurysm and preventing recanalization. The bioactive coils are designed to augment the healing response and promote collagen synthesis, thus reducing the risk of coil compaction and aneurysm recanalization. They are not intended to replace dense packing of the aneurysm, which is necessary to resist the impact of blood flow on the aneurysm. Elimination of the water-hammer effect of blood flow is crucial to create a milieu for the healing process to be effective. In this article, we review our current understanding of aneurysm growth, the mechanisms of tissue scarring, the effect of biodegradable polymers on healing, and the experiments supporting the augmented healing response by Matrix coils. We hope to stimulate new ideas and encourage the development of new generations of bioactive coils for the further advancement of endovascular treatment of aneurysms. Finally, we present some typical cases and the UCLA experience to illustrate the biologic effect of Matrix coils. The long-term efficacy data on Matrix coils

---

* Corresponding author.
E-mail address: lfeng@mednet.ucla.edu (L. Feng).

are not available at this point and are thus beyond the scope of this article. Because fusiform aneurysms are usually treated with parent vessel occlusion, the discussions in this article only involve saccular aneurysms.

Yin and yang of aneurysm growth: injury versus healing

Understanding the cellular and molecular pathogenesis of intracranial aneurysms is essential for developing new treatment strategies. Disrupted internal elastic lamina is the pathologic hallmark of intracranial aneurysms. The blood vessel wall contains intima, media, and adventitia. Intima is lined by endothelial cells on the luminal surface and consists of extracellular matrix and a few smooth muscle cells. The internal elastic lamina, which contains collagen type III and elastin, separates intima from media. Smooth muscle cells and collagen fibers comprise most media. The intracranial arteries have relatively thin media and little adventitia compared with coronary arteries of similar size. Injury and repair are constantly at play in the vascular wall and may lead to various types of vascular diseases, including aneurysms.

Risk factors for intracranial aneurysms and subarachnoid hemorrhage

A genetic defect in the collagen or extracellular matrix synthesis can lead to weakness in the blood vessels. According to several epidemiology studies [8–10], the first-degree relatives of patients with intracranial aneurysms have a higher incidence of intracranial aneurysms than the normal population, suggesting the presence of hereditary factors in the development of intracranial aneurysms. A recent Finnish study identified 346 families with intracranial aneurysms: an autosomal recessive inheritance pattern was noted in 57.2% of the families, 36.4% of the families showed autosomal dominance, and another 5.5% of the families were consistent with autosomal dominance with incomplete penetrance [9]. These studies support the existence of major genetic defects in at least a subpopulation of patients with intracranial aneurysms. The associations of aneurysms with inherited diseases [11], particularly polycystic kidney disease [12,13] and Ehlers-Danlos syndrome [14], have been reported; however, the denominators of these observations are not known, and

a prospective study failed to establish a statistically significant association between polycystic kidney disease and intracranial aneurysms [15]. So far, no candidate gene has been convincingly identified. The potential underlying gene mutations may interact or require additional environmental factors as well. It is also difficult to identify all family members with intracranial aneurysms for linkage analysis. The improvement of noninvasive imaging techniques to detect intracranial aneurysms may facilitate future genetic studies.

Cigarette smoking and hypertension are exogenous factors that have been associated with the development of intracranial aneurysms and subarachnoid hemorrhage [16–19]. Heavy alcohol consumption has been associated with aneurysmal subarachnoid hemorrhage in case-control studies [20,21], but this association has not been convincingly proven in longitudinal studies [22,23]. Although many case series and the cooperative study showed a higher incidence of subarachnoid hemorrhage in women than in men [24], male preponderance has been observed in some geographic areas [8]. Population-based studies are required to establish gender further as an independent risk factor [25].

Vascular injury and repair

Repetitive vascular injury leads to chronic inflammation and continuous remodeling in the vessel wall. Leukocytes, particularly monocytes, infiltrate into the vessel wall and secrete various degradative enzymes, including many matrix metalloproteinases (MMPs), causing destruction of the extracellular matrix. Conversely, these inflammatory cells release several cytokines and growth factors to promote the infiltration of macrophages and proliferation of smooth muscle cells and fibroblasts. Macrophages engulf the degraded extracellular matrix and cellular debris, whereas smooth muscle cells and fibroblasts synthesize new collagen and elastin. This destruction and rebuilding process ebbs and flows and is modulated by the endothelial cells, which sense the physical and chemical milieu of the blood vessel. This process is collectively called vascular remodeling and forms the basis for the development of many vascular diseases.

Cigarette smoking and hypertension, established risk factors for chronic vascular injury leading to the development of atherosclerosis, can predispose patients to intracranial aneurysms as well. Cigarette smoking increases the oxidative stress in the vessel wall and induces an inflammatory response, which can undermine the structural integrity of blood vessels [26,27]. Hypertension increases the mechanical stress on the vessel wall and induces vascular remodeling [28,29]. In response to excessive mechanical stretch, the activities of MMPs are increased, destroying the old extracellular matrix scaffold to allow the synthesis and organization of new extracellular matrix [30,31].

Intracranial aneurysms frequently arise from bifurcation sites, where the turbulent flow generates high shear stress. High shear stress can induce the remodeling process involving the destruction of old cellular components and extracellular matrix structure and the synthesis of a vessel segment adaptive to the rheotology [32,33]. Stagnation may also occur in the shoulder of turbulent flow, resulting in oxidative stress and the induction of nitric oxide, leading to degenerative changes in the vessel wall [34]. Inhibition of nitric oxide synthase has been shown to attenuate early aneurysmal changes and aneurysm formation in a rat model [35]. The water-hammer effect exerted on the aneurysm inflow zone can result in mechanical injury and continuous growth of the aneurysm [36,37].

Endothelial denudation, infiltration of inflammatory cells, smooth muscle proliferation, destruction of extracellular matrix, and apoptosis, the hallmarks of vascular remodeling, have all been observed in histologic specimens of intracranial aneurysms [38–41]. Increased activities of MMPs have been observed in aneurysm walls [40,42,43]. Although this process frequently leads to atherosclerosis and intimal hyperplasia [30], deficient synthesis of the extracellular matrix and failed regulation of cellular proliferation and the overproduction of degradative enzymes can all result in inadequate repair, leaving an anatomic defect in the vessel wall. The enhanced vessel wall destruction can thus interact with a genetic or acquired deficiency in extracellular matrix synthesis to create an aneurysm (Fig. 1). Once a small defect occurs in the vessel wall, the altered flow dynamic may prompt additional vascular injury, a constant remodeling reaction, and repetition of the same deficient repair, leading to the gradual growth of the aneurysm.

Because of this dynamic process in the vessel wall, treatment of an aneurysm can be achieved by promoting a healing response to increase smooth muscle proliferation and extracellular matrix deposition. This healing process results in thickening of the intima and media to counteract the hemodynamic stress and prevent the aneurysm from further growth or rupture.

Organization of thrombus and aneurysm recanalization

Aneurysm recanalization may occur immediately after embolization or during thrombus organization or later remodeling of the aneurysm neck. During embolization, stasis and thrombogenicity of GDCs promote thrombosis in the lumen of an aneurysm. In the meantime, the thrombolytic pathway is activated and may dissolve part of the thrombus. Because the coil mass and stasis hinder the access of plasminogen and plasmin to the newly formed thrombus, the dynamic process usually tilts toward thrombosis. Recanalization of the aneurysm from thrombolysis is thus only a theoretic concern unless the aneurysm is severely underpacked or the patient is placed on anticoagulation therapy. The newly formed fibrin meshwork in the thrombus continues to polymerize and becomes densely compacted and resistant to thrombolysis within the first 24 hours. The remaining thrombus undergoes organization to become a scar or partially recanalized through neovascularity. Coil compaction may occur during thrombus organization, which takes a few weeks to complete, resulting in partial recanalization of the aneurysm. Once a tough fibrous scar forms, the coil masses are fixed in space and less likely to compact. Even after a stable fibrous tissue forms, the remodeling process can continue for many years in a fashion similar to de novo growth of an aneurysm if the original vascular insult remains uncorrected and the turbulent flow at the aneurysm neck maintains significant mechanical stress on the vessel wall.

Cellular mechanisms of thrombus organization

As the first step of thrombus organization, mesenchymal cells infiltrate into the thrombus to form granulation tissue. Leukocytes and platelets trapped in the thrombus release degradative enzymes to break down the fibrin meshwork. If the thrombus is large, as is usually the case in underpacked large aneurysms, the center of the thrombus may be liquefied, allowing coil compaction to occur. Endothelial precursor cells migrate into the thrombus and coalesce into a capillary network, which connects with the blood flow and brings in more inflammatory cells. Macrophages

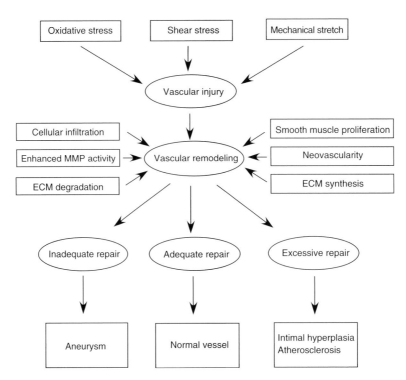

Fig. 1. Vascular remodeling. Oxidative stress caused by cigarette smoking, excessive mechanical stretch of the arterial wall in patients with hypertension, and increased shear stress at vascular bifurcation points can all lead to vascular injury, triggering vascular remodeling, which involves further destruction and rebuilding of the vessel wall. Infiltration of inflammatory cells and increased activity of matrix metalloproteinase (MMP) activities remove cellular debris and dissolve the old extracellular matrix (ECM) scaffold. Smooth muscle proliferation and neovascularization take place at the site of vascular remodeling, followed by the synthesis of new ECM. The integrity of the vessel wall is restored with adequate repair. When repair is inadequate, an anatomic defect may result, leading to the formation of an aneurysm. Conversely, excessive repair can contribute to intimal hyperplasia and atherosclerosis.

engulf the fibrin degradation products and cellular debris as fibroblasts and smooth muscle cells proliferate and synthesize new extracellular matrix, including collagen, fibronectin, and elastin. Smooth muscle cells are the major cellular component of neointima, which covers the neck of an embolized aneurysm. Their activation and proliferation are critical for adequate healing of the aneurysm [44]. The thrombus is gradually replaced by fibrous scar tissue, which is strengthened by extracellular matrix proteins, particularly collagen fibers, rendering the scar tissue resistant to the flow dynamic effect at the aneurysm neck. If the synthesis of extracellular matrix proteins is reduced, the scar tissue may contract, causing additional coil compaction and aneurysm recanalization. In addition, the capillary network, which usually disappears in the later stage of the healing reaction, may

enlarge and become incorporated into the parent vessel, resulting in partial or even complete recanalization.

Because healing is intimately related to destruction, promoting the healing response can be a double-edged sword. Increased cellular infiltrate at the early stage of the healing response can result in rapid softening and destruction of the fibrin thrombus, thus facilitating coil compaction. Angiogenesis enhances the healing response but risks recanalization at a later stage. Adequate packing of the aneurysm is crucial in preventing recanalization by limiting early thrombolysis, reducing the size of the thrombus, and modifying flow dynamics at the aneurysm neck. Modulating the healing response, particularly the synthesis of extracellular matrix proteins, may promote the formation of dense scar tissue to reduce the risk of recanalization.

Extracellular matrix synthesis

The regulation of extracellular matrix synthesis is a complex process involving many cytokines, including transforming growth factor-β (TGFβ), connective tissue growth factor (CTGF), tissue necrosis factor-α (TNFα), and interferon-γ (IFNγ) [45]. TGFβ induces fibroblasts to synthesize and contract extracellular matrix and has long been regarded as a key mediator of the healing response [46]. It also suppresses the transcription of MMPs, preventing the degradation of newly synthesized extracellular matrix. TGFβ is synthesized as a latent precursor complexed with latent TGFβ binding protein and covalently linked to the extracellular matrix [47]. Proteolytic cleavage of latent TGFβ precursor by metalloproteinases, which promote matrix degradation, activates the healing response through TGFβ. Other TGFβ activators include thrombospondin-1 (TSP-1) and integrin $\alpha_v\beta_6$. TSP-1 modulates cell adhesion, angiogenesis, and reconstruction of matrix. Transgenic mice with TSP-1 knock-out share many phenotypes with TGFβ null mutants [48]. Without integrin β_6, the transgenic mice are protected against lung fibrosis when treated with the profibrotic drug bleomycin [49]. CTGF is synthesized in the endothelial cells in response to TGFβ and is thought to carry out the downstream effects TGFβ on fibroblasts [50]. TNFα and IFNγ are the major inhibitors of extracellular matrix synthesis. TNFα released by macrophages interferes with signal transduction of TGFβ, thus suppressing the synthesis of extracellular matrix genes [51,52]. IFNγ is made by T cells and inhibits collagen production through its signal transduction pathway [53].

The complexity of these interwoven regulatory mechanisms makes it impossible to use a single cytokine or growth factor to promote a desirable healing response in aneurysms. Conversely, the counteracting factors maintain the healing response under strict control, reducing the risk of parent vessel occlusion by exaggerated fibrosis.

Modulation of healing response in animal models of cerebral aneurysm

Ever since the introduction of GDCs, various modifications of GDCs have been studied in animal models to promote the healing response in aneurysms. Based on the agents used, these modifications can be categorized as extracellular matrix proteins, growth factors and/or cytokines, and bioactive polymers.

Coils coated with extracellular matrix proteins

Extracellular matrix proteins, including type 1 collagen, fibronectin, vitronectin, fibrinogen, and laminin, have been used to coat GDCs with ion-implantation technology [54]. The protein-coated coils behaved similarly to plain GDCs in their mechanical properties when used to embolize experimental side-wall aneurysms in swine [55]. These modified coils demonstrated a faster and enhanced cellular response in the aneurysm body and dome and the formation of a fibrous and endothelialized covering of the aneurysm neck. Favorable anatomic and histologic results were also obtained with collagen-based coils in a rabbit model [56]. Because these extracellular matrix proteins are highly thrombogenic, it is not clear whether the enhanced healing response is secondary to increased thrombosis or direct integration of these extracellular matrix proteins. Nevertheless, the extracellular matrix proteins provide an excellent substrate for the adhesion and migration of inflammatory cells and endothelial cells, which may contribute to the faster and stronger inflammatory response in the aneurysm and neointima formation at the aneurysm neck.

Coils coated with cytokines and/or growth factors

Given its critical role in regulating extracellular matrix synthesis, TGFβ is a prime candidate for coating bioactive coils. When TGFβ-coated coils were compared with plain platinum coils in a rabbit model of aneurysm, increased thickness of the neointima at the aneurysm neck was noted 2 weeks after embolization [57]. The difference decreased at 6 weeks, suggesting that TGFβ coating may accelerate cellular proliferation and production of extracellular matrix at the coil-lumen interface. Because this experiment was performed with significant underpacking of the aneurysm to study the interaction between the coil surface and surrounding tissue and there was no angiographic follow-up, it remains unknown if TGFβ coating has any effect on obliterating aneurysms or preventing recanalization. To determine if TGFβ can stimulate neointima formation at the aneurysm neck, Desfaits et al [58] delivered gelatin sponges soaked with TGFβ into experimental porcine and canine aneurysms. They found that a high dose of TGFβ (600 ng) significantly increased neointima thickness at the neck of porcine aneurysms, whereas a low dose of TGFβ had no effect. Surprisingly, no difference was seen in canine aneurysms. Similarly, the homodimer of platelet-derived growth factor B subunits (PDGF-BB) or platelet extract that contains PDGF increased neointima thickness in porcine aneurysms but failed to improve healing of canine aneurysms [58,59]. The authors attributed this discrepancy between porcine and canine aneurysms to deficient thrombosis in the canine model and the consequent lack of matrix support for cell migration and proliferation. If the thrombus is dissolved by the thrombolytic pathway before organization, there would not be any substrate for the activity of these growth factors.

Because angiogenesis accompanies the organization of thrombus, Abraham et al [51] tested the hypothesis that vascular endothelial growth factor (VEGF), which stimulates endothelial cell proliferation, could enhance fibrosis and obliteration of aneurysms when released from GDCs. These authors created a rat aneurysm model by ligating the common carotid artery and inserted coil segments without coating or coated with type I collagen or type I collagen and human recombinant VEGF into the blind-ended sac. They found increased wall thickness with VEGF-coated coils and an enhanced cellular reaction on the surface of VEGF-coated coils.

Basic fibroblast growth factor (bFGF) has been demonstrated to stimulate the proliferation and migration of endothelial cells, smooth muscle cells, and fibroblasts as well as the production of type 1 collagen by smooth muscle cells and fibroblasts [60]. Because of its short-half life in circulation, direct application of bFGF to an aneurysm is ineffective. Hatano et al [61] developed a polyethylene terephthalate (PET) fiber coil coated with gelatin hydrogel containing bFGF to release bFGF slowly into the aneurysm. They tested this coil in a rabbit venous pouch aneurysm model and demonstrated increased fibrosis, neointima formation, and closure of the aneurysm neck using bFGF-eluting gelatin hydrogel PET coils compared with gelatin hydrogel PET coils without bFGF. This prototype of drug-eluting coils opens a new dimension to modulate the healing process in aneurysms.

Similar to the delivery of growth factors, coils have also been used as a platform to deliver cellular grafts that secrete growth factors or are expected to integrate into the vessel wall during the healing process. When fibroblasts transformed with human bFGF gene were introduced into rat carotid arteries using a GDC as the carrier, increased fibroblast proliferation was observed in the vessel wall at 14 days [62]. At 35 days, there was an increase in fibroblast proliferation and collagen synthesis. Further studies showed that fibroblasts grown on GDCs and introduced into aneurysms in a rabbit elastase model can remain viable and proliferate in the vicinity of coils [63]. Progressive cellular proliferation and increased fibrosis were observed in the aneurysms treated with cellular grafts compared with those treated with GDCs alone.

The delivery of growth factors and cellular grafts are higher levels of modulation of the healing process than the introduction of extracellular matrix proteins. Nevertheless, many cytokines and growth factors are involved in the healing process. Which growth factor or combination of growth factors is the most effective treatment remains unknown. The timing and dosing of these growth factors require further studies as well. Cellular grafts may have the advantage of sensing the needs for these growth factors and releasing them at the appropriate time and in the appropriate amount. Nonetheless, genetic manipulation of cellular grafts may be required to activate these cells, and the creation of an appropriate milieu may be necessary for these cells to carry out the desired healing function instead of destruction or overzealous cellular proliferation and extracellular matrix synthesis, leading to parent vessel stenosis. GDCs can serve as a drug-eluting and cellular graft platform, facilitating the delivery, visualization, and controlled release of therapeutic agents.

Matrix coils

Although many of these extracellular matrix proteins and cytokines have shown beneficial effects in promoting a healing response in experimental aneurysms, none of them have passed the preclinical stage. As pointed out earlier, the healing response involves several processes that are influenced by different extracellular proteins and cytokines. Exaggeration of an individual process in the healing response, whether that is cellular proliferation, angiogenesis, or extracellular matrix synthesis, may be counterproductive and increase the risk of recanalization or parent vessel stenosis. In addition, the toxicity and long-term safety of these extracellular matrix proteins or growth factors in human beings, particularly inside blood vessels, have not been adequately studied. The regulatory hurdle for moving these agents to the clinical stage is thus high.

Furthermore, the cellular and molecular mechanisms of aneurysm development and the healing response after embolization have just begun to be elucidated. Future studies are likely to identify better therapeutic targets and better therapeutic agents for the modulation of the healing response.

In contrast, bioabsorbable polymers, such as polyglycolic acid and polyglycolic/poly-L-lactic acid copolymer (PLGA), have been well studied and widely used in tissue engineering applications [64–66]. They can regulate the healing response in the adjacent tissues during their biologic degradation: the faster the degradation, the stronger is the tissue reaction [67,68]. The degradation rate of PLGA can be altered by changing the composition of lactic and glycolic acids. A high concentration of lactic acid renders the polymer resistant to degradation enzymes [69]. This property can thus be used to control the healing response after coil embolization.

To investigate the cellular responses to different compositions of PLGA, Murayama et al [70] placed PLGA at lactide/glycolic acid ratios of 85:15, 75:25, 65:35, and 50:50 into 16 experimental aneurysms in eight swine. They found that PLGA with faster degradation rates (ie, lower lactide content [65:35 and 50:50]) induced more mature collagen deposition and fibrosis in the sac and neck of aneurysms than polymers that are more resistant to degradation. The levels of collagen formation were linearly correlated to the degradation rates of PLGA polymers. This experiment demonstrated the feasibility of using bioabsorbable polymers to accelerate the healing response in aneurysms and paved the road for the manufacture of Matrix coils.

Matrix coils comprise an inner core of plain platinum coils and an outer layer of PLGA, which is affixed to the platinum core by heating. The platinum core provides radiopacity and coil shape memory. The size and physical properties of Matrix coils are similar to those of GDCs; however, the presence of PLGA on the outside of the platinum core does increase friction during coil delivery.

Murayama et al [71,72] used a swine aneurysm model to demonstrate accelerated wound healing in aneurysms treated with Matrix coils compared with plain GDCs. They created 24 aneurysms in 12 animals. One aneurysm in each animal was randomly chosen to be embolized with Matrix coils, and the other aneurysm was embolized with plain GDCs as a control. The aneurysms treated with Matrix coils were intentionally underpacked

to study the healing response, whereas the other aneurysms were packed with GDCs as densely as possible. Angiographic follow-up obtained at 14 days after embolization showed a gap between the coil mass and the contrast-filled parent vessel in 75% of aneurysms treated with Matrix coils, suggesting neointima formation at the aneurysm neck; none of the aneurysms treated with regular GDCs had this finding. At 3 months, evidence of neointima formation was observed in all aneurysms treated with Matrix coils but in none of the aneurysms treated with regular GDCs. Histologic examination revealed a higher grade of cellular response around the coils, lower percentage of unorganized thrombus, and thicker neointima in the neck of aneurysms treated with Matrix coils than of those treated with regular GDCs. The thick neointima remained 3 months after embolization. In addition, there was no incidence of parent vessel stenosis or thrombosis. It should be noted that Matrix coils have less thrombogenicity than standard GDCs; thus, their action is not based on promotion of thrombosis within the aneurysm. Retraction of the aneurysm was observed at 3 months after treatment, suggesting the possibility of reducing mass effect after embolization. These results showed great promise of Matrix coils to enhance the healing response in aneurysms and reduce the risk of recanalization.

Hydrocoils

To improve packing of the aneurysm, which is another important factor in preventing recanalization, coils coated with expandable hydrogels (Hydrocoils; Microvention Inc., Aliso Viejo, California) have been developed and approved by US Food and Drug Administration (FDA) for clinical use. Hydrocoils consists of platinum coils coated with a synthetic polyalcohol, which can swell to nine times its original volume when placed into blood. The hydration process is slow enough to allow deployment and retraction of the coil for at least 5 minutes. Animal studies in a rabbit aneurysm model showed that Hydrocoils can improve aneurysm filling from the historical 20% to 30% with standard GDCs to a mean of 68% [73]. Hydrogel was biologically inert and did not stimulate an inflammatory reaction or healing response. Poor organized thrombus remained in the aneurysm after 14 days, and the aneurysm neck was covered with a thin fibrous layer as often seen in aneurysms treated with standard GDCs. Initial clinical experience with Hydrocoils confirmed improved packing of aneurysms from 32% in aneurysms treated with standard GDCs to 72% in aneurysms treated with Hydrocoils [74]. Although Hydrocoils have no effect on the healing response, improved packing of aneurysms, particularly in large and giant aneurysms, can have significant beneficial effects on preventing recanalization.

Preliminary clinical experience with Matrix coils

Since the first patient received Matrix coils in June 2002, a total of 150 saccular aneurysms in 140 patients have been treated with Matrix coils at UCLA. These patients include 116 women and 24 men, with an average age of 57 ± 1 years. Fifty-three patients presented with acute subarachnoid hemorrhage, 14 patients had subarachnoid hemorrhage but came to our service after the acute phase, and the other 77 patients had unruptured aneurysms. Among the patients with unruptured aneurysms, seven were symptomatic from mass effects, and the other 70 patients had incidental aneurysms. The distribution of these aneurysms is shown in Table 1. One hundred eighteen aneurysms were in the anterior circulation, including 32 posterior communicating artery aneurysms and 29 anterior communicating artery aneurysms, the two most common sites. Thirty-three aneurysms were in the posterior circulation, including 20 basilar artery aneurysms. There were 99 (66.0%) small (≤10 mm), 50 (33.3%) large (11–25 mm), and 1 (0.7%) giant (>25 mm) aneurysms. Sixty-nine of these aneurysms (46.0%) had a small neck, and 81 (54.0%) had a wide neck. A total of 157 embolization procedures were performed on these aneurysms. Complete obliteration of the aneurysm was achieved at the end of the procedure in 60 (38.2%) cases, and 14 (8.9%) aneurysms were partially coiled. The remaining aneurysms (52.9%) had small neck remnants. The high percentage of neck remnants may be related to the increased sensitivity of using a three-dimensional rotational angiogram to detect small neck remnants; most of these aneurysms would have been considered completely obliterated by planar angiography. There were six intraoperative ruptures and eight thromboembolic complications. Parent vessel narrowing after embolization occurred in only 1 patient, who had a small loop of coil herniating into the parent vessel.

Eighty patients with 90 aneurysms have had follow-up angiograms, with an average interval of 8 ± 0.6 months. Based on preliminary analysis of

Table 1
Distribution of aneurysms in Matrix coil series at the University of California at Los Angeles

Location	Number	Percentage
Anterior circulation		
Anterior choroidal	3	2.0%
Anterior communicating	29	19.3%
Cavernous carotid	7	4.7%
Carotid cave	10	6.7%
Internal carotid bifurcation	3	2.0%
Middle cerebral	7	4.7%
Ophthalmic	15	10.0%
Posterior communicating	32	21.3%
Superior hypophyseal	11	7.3%
Posterior circulation		
Anterior inferior cerebellar	1	0.7%
Basilar	20	13.3%
Posterior cerebral	3	2.0%
Posterior inferior cerebellar	3	2.0%
Superior cerebellar	6	4.0%
Total	150	

the data, 21 patients showed progressive thrombosis and reduction of the residual neck, suggesting successful healing of the aneurysms. A white-collar sign was observed in several cases (Fig. 2), indicating the formation of thick fibrous intima at the aneurysm neck. Most aneurysms remained stable during follow-up. Durable results were obtained in many large and wide-neck aneurysms, which are at high risk of recanalization (Fig. 3). Twelve aneurysms (13.3%) showed significant recanalization, requiring further treatment. Only 1 patient had repeat subarachnoid hemorrhage after embolization. This patient had a basilar artery aneurysm with a wide neck and received dome protection during the acute phase of her first subarachnoid hemorrhage. She rebled in 2 months, before scheduled definitive therapy with stent assistance.

Patient selection bias could have masked some of the beneficial effects of Matrix coils. Matrix coils were more likely to be used in large and wide-neck aneurysms, which are more likely to recanalize than small aneurysms. The percentage of large aneurysms in this case series is almost twice as high as in our previously published series [4]. Multivariate analysis is thus required to draw a conclusion. In addition, the friction of Matrix coils could have contributed to underpacking of the aneurysms. Despite its healing effect, the strong water-hammer effect of blood flow can still compact the coils in partially coiled aneurysms. The follow-up period is still too short to assess the

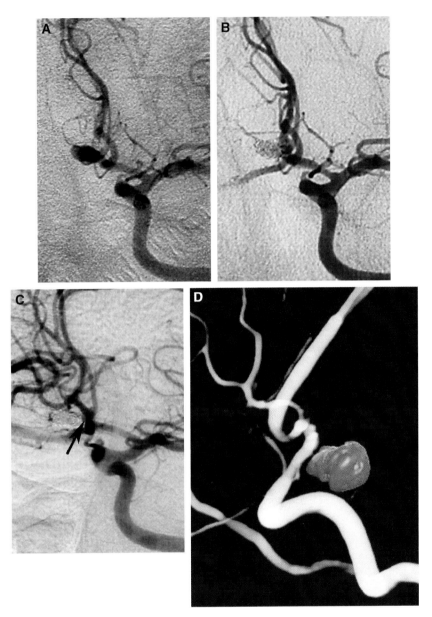

Fig. 2.   White-collar sign. (*A*) This patient presents with a ruptured anterior communicating artery aneurysm. (*B*) At the end of Matrix coil embolization, the dome of the aneurysm is obliterated but there is still a small amount of contrast filling at the neck of the aneurysm. (*C*) Follow-up angiogram 3 months later reveals complete occlusion of the aneurysm neck. The coil mass is separated from the parent vessel by a thin white line (*arrow*), the white-collar sign, suggesting fibrous neointima at the aneurysm neck. (*D*) Three-dimensional angiography illustrates another example of the white-collar sign at 13 months of follow-up in a patient with a ruptured posterior communicating artery aneurysm. The coil mass is depicted in red.

long-term clinical outcome and rebleed rate of Matrix coil embolization.

In our experience, patients with unruptured aneurysms sometimes develop headaches in the first few days after embolization with Matrix coils. These headaches usually subside after 1 week and respond to nonsteroidal anti-inflammatory drugs or rapid-taper steroid therapy, suggesting that they are related to inflammation incited by the Matrix coils. Whether anti-inflammatory therapy interferes with healing or not remains unknown.

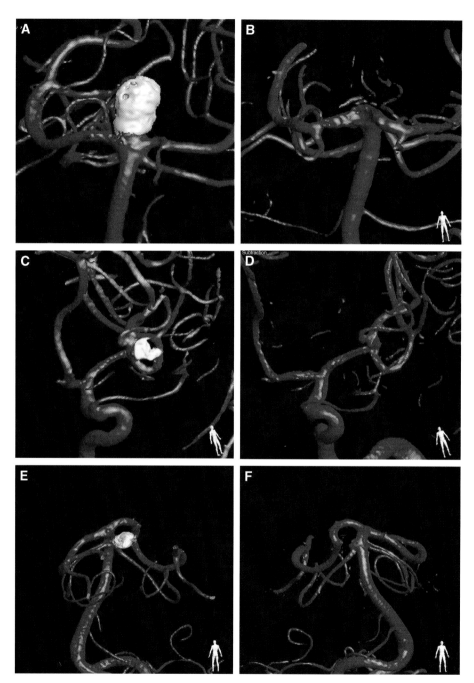

Fig. 3. Durable Matrix coil embolization of aneurysms. (*A*) Anterior-posterior projection of a three-dimensional rotational angiogram shows a completely occluded wide-neck basilar tip aneurysm at 14 months of follow-up. The coil mass is depicted in white. (*B*) After subtraction of the white coil mass, the angiogram shows no evidence of a residual neck. (*C*) Left anterior oblique projection of a three-dimensional rotation angiogram reveals near-complete obliteration of a wide-neck left middle cerebral artery bifurcation aneurysm at 18 months of follow-up. The subtracted image is shown in *D*. (*E*) Twelve months after embolization, this wide-neck right superior cerebellar artery aneurysm remains completely occluded (posterior-anterior projection). (*F*) The subtracted image (anterior-posterior projection) shows preservation of the right superior cerebellar artery.

In summary, Matrix coils are designed to promote healing and reduce recanalization in well-embolized aneurysms; they are not meant to replace dense packing of aneurysms. Although we have observed evidence of a healing response in our preliminary clinical experience using Matrix coils, the benefit of Matrix coils is not dramatic and requires further studies for confirmation. Friction of the coils may limit dense packing of aneurysms. For this reason, we usually use Matrix coils as framing or filling coils and use regular GDCs as the last few finishing coils. Nonetheless, the Matrix coil is the first step in the future direction of improving endovascular treatment of aneurysms. Although it may be tempting to conduct a clinical trial to prove the efficacy of Matrix coils, resources can probably be better used in developing new generations of bioactive coils based on an understanding of the molecular pathogenesis of aneurysms and on the cellular and molecular mechanisms of tissue healing.

References

[1] Guglielmi G, Vinuela F, Sepetka I, et al. Electro-thrombosis of saccular aneurysms via endovascular approach. Part 1: electrochemical basis, technique, and experimental results. J Neurosurg 1991;75:1–7.

[2] Guglielmi G, Vinuela F, Dion J, et al. Electrothrombosis of saccular aneurysms via endovascular approach. Part 2: preliminary clinical experience. J Neurosurg 1991;75:8–14.

[3] Molyneux A, Kerr R, Stratton I, et al. International Subarachnoid Aneurysm Trial (ISAT) of neurosurgical clipping versus endovascular coiling in 2143 patients with ruptured intracranial aneurysms: a randomised trial. Lancet 2002;360:1267–74.

[4] Murayama Y, Nien YL, Duckwiler G, et al. Guglielmi detachable coil embolization of cerebral aneurysms: 11 years' experience. J Neurosurg 2003;98:959–66.

[5] Byrne JV, Sohn MJ, Molyneux AJ, et al. Five-year experience in using coil embolization for ruptured intracranial aneurysms: outcomes and incidence of late rebleeding. J Neurosurg 1999;90:656–63.

[6] Ng P, Khangure MS, Phatouros CC, et al. Endovascular treatment of intracranial aneurysms with Guglielmi detachable coils: analysis of midterm angiographic and clinical outcomes. Stroke 2002;33:210–7.

[7] Lempert TE, Malek AM, Halbach VV, et al. Endovascular treatment of ruptured posterior circulation cerebral aneurysms. Clinical and angiographic outcomes. Stroke 2000;31:100–10.

[8] Ronkainen A, Hernesniemi J, Puranen M, et al. Familial intracranial aneurysms. Lancet 1997;349:380–4.

[9] Wills S, Ronkainen A, van der Voet M, et al. Familial intracranial aneurysms: an analysis of 346 multiplex Finnish families. Stroke 2003;34:1370–4.

[10] Raaymakers TW. Aneurysms in relatives of patients with subarachnoid hemorrhage: frequency and risk factors. MARS Study Group. Magnetic Resonance Angiography in Relatives of patients with Subarachnoid hemorrhage. Neurology 1999;53:982–8.

[11] Nekrysh SY. Association between heritable connective tissue disorders and intracranial aneurysms. Surg Neurol 2000;54:77–8.

[12] Poutasse EF, Gardner WJ, McCormack CL. Polycystic kidney disease and intracranial aneurysm. JAMA 1954;154:741–4.

[13] Schievink WI, Torres VE, Piepgras DG, et al. Saccular intracranial aneurysms in autosomal dominant polycystic kidney disease. J Am Soc Nephrol 1992;3:88–95.

[14] Rubinstein MK, Cohen NH. Ehlers-Danlos syndrome associated with multiple intracranial aneurysms. Neurology 1964;14:125–32.

[15] Chapman AB, Rubinstein D, Hughes R, et al. Intracranial aneurysms in autosomal dominant polycystic kidney disease. N Engl J Med 1992;327:916–20.

[16] Bell BA, Symon L. Smoking and subarachnoid haemorrhage. BMJ 1979;1:577–8.

[17] Juvela S. Natural history of unruptured intracranial aneurysms: risks for aneurysm formation, growth, and rupture. Acta Neurochir Suppl (Wien) 2002;82:27–30.

[18] Kissela BM, Sauerbeck L, Woo D, et al. Subarachnoid hemorrhage: a preventable disease with a heritable component. Stroke 2002;33:1321–6.

[19] Weir BK, Kongable GL, Kassell NF, et al. Cigarette smoking as a cause of aneurysmal subarachnoid hemorrhage and risk for vasospasm: a report of the Cooperative Aneurysm Study. J Neurosurg 1998;89:405–11.

[20] Longstreth WT Jr, Nelson LM, Koepsell TD, et al. Cigarette smoking, alcohol use, and subarachnoid hemorrhage. Stroke 1992;23:1242–9.

[21] Juvela S, Hillbom M, Numminen H, et al. Cigarette smoking and alcohol consumption as risk factors for aneurysmal subarachnoid hemorrhage. Stroke 1993;24:639–46.

[22] Donahue RP, Abbott RD, Reed DM, et al. Alcohol and hemorrhagic stroke. The Honolulu Heart Program. JAMA 1986;255:2311–4.

[23] Stampfer MJ, Colditz GA, Willett WC, et al. A prospective study of moderate alcohol consumption and the risk of coronary disease and stroke in women. N Engl J Med 1988;319:267–73.

[24] Kongable GL, Lanzino G, Germanson TP, et al. Gender-related differences in aneurysmal subarachnoid hemorrhage. J Neurosurg 1996;84:43–8.

[25] Fischer T, Johnsen SP, Pedersen L, et al. Seasonal variation in hospitalization and case fatality of subarachnoid hemorrhage—a nationwide Danish study on 9,367 patients. Neuroepidemiology 2005;24:32–7.

[26] Burke A, Fitzgerald GA. Oxidative stress and smoking-induced vascular injury. Prog Cardiovasc Dis 2003;46:79–90.

[27] Ambrose JA, Barua RS. The pathophysiology of cigarette smoking and cardiovascular disease: an update. J Am Coll Cardiol 2004;43:1731–7.

[28] Lehoux S, Lemarie CA, Esposito B, et al. Pressure-induced matrix metalloproteinase-9 contributes to early hypertensive remodeling. Circulation 2004;109:1041–7.

[29] Shaw A, Xu Q. Biomechanical stress-induced signaling in smooth muscle cells: an update. Curr Vasc Pharmacol 2003;1:41–58.

[30] Galis ZS, Khatri JJ. Matrix metalloproteinases in vascular remodeling and atherogenesis: the good, the bad, and the ugly. Circ Res 2002;90:251–62.

[31] Bradley JM, Kelley MJ, Zhu X, et al. Effects of mechanical stretching on trabecular matrix metalloproteinases. Invest Ophthalmol Vis Sci 2001;42:1505–13.

[32] Hoshina K, Sho E, Sho M, et al. Wall shear stress and strain modulate experimental aneurysm cellularity. J Vasc Surg 2003;37:1067–74.

[33] Rossitti S, Lofgren J. Vascular dimensions of the cerebral arteries follow the principle of minimum work. Stroke 1993;24:371–7.

[34] Nakatani H, Hashimoto N, Kang Y, et al. Cerebral blood flow patterns at major vessel bifurcations and aneurysms in rats. J Neurosurg 1991;74:258–62.

[35] Fukuda S, Hashimoto N, Naritomi H, et al. Prevention of rat cerebral aneurysm formation by inhibition of nitric oxide synthase. Circulation 2000;101:2532–8.

[36] Tateshima S, Vinuela F, Villablanca JP, et al. Three-dimensional blood flow analysis in a wide-necked internal carotid artery-ophthalmic artery aneurysm. J Neurosurg 2003;99:526–33.

[37] Kwan ES, Heilman CB, Shucart WA, et al. Enlargement of basilar artery aneurysms following balloon occlusion—"water-hammer effect." Report of two cases. J Neurosurg 1991;75:963–8.

[38] Hara A, Yoshimi N, Mori H. Evidence for apoptosis in human intracranial aneurysms. Neurol Res 1998;20:127–30.

[39] Chyatte D, Bruno G, Desai S, et al. Inflammation and intracranial aneurysms. Neurosurgery 1999;45:1137–46; discussion, 1146–7.

[40] Bruno G, Todor R, Lewis I, et al. Vascular extracellular matrix remodeling in cerebral aneurysms. J Neurosurg 1998;89:431–40.

[41] Nakajima N, Nagahiro S, Sano T, et al. Phenotypic modulation of smooth muscle cells in human cerebral aneurysmal walls. Acta Neuropathol (Berl) 2000;100:475–80.

[42] Chyatte D, Lewis I. Gelatinase activity and the occurrence of cerebral aneurysms. Stroke 1997;28:799–804.

[43] Gaetani P, Rodriguez y Baena R, Tartara F, et al. Metalloproteases and intracranial vascular lesions. Neurol Res 1999;21:385–90.

[44] Raymond J, Venne D, Allas S, et al. Healing mechanisms in experimental aneurysms. I. Vascular smooth muscle cells and neointima formation. J Neuroradiol 1999;26:7–20.

[45] Leask A, Abraham DJ. TGF-beta signaling and the fibrotic response. FASEB J 2004;18:816–27.

[46] Massague J. TGF-beta signal transduction. Annu Rev Biochem 1998;67:753–91.

[47] Annes JP, Munger JS, Rifkin DB. Making sense of latent TGFbeta activation. J Cell Sci 2003;116:217–24.

[48] Crawford SE, Stellmach V, Murphy-Ullrich JE, et al. Thrombospondin-1 is a major activator of TGF-beta1 in vivo. Cell 1998;93:1159–70.

[49] Munger JS, Huang X, Kawakatsu H, et al. The integrin alpha v beta 6 binds and activates latent TGF beta 1: a mechanism for regulating pulmonary inflammation and fibrosis. Cell 1999;96:319–28.

[50] Grotendorst GR. Connective tissue growth factor: a mediator of TGF-beta action on fibroblasts. Cytokine Growth Factor Rev 1997;8:171–9.

[51] Abraham DJ, Shiwen X, Black CM, et al. Tumor necrosis factor alpha suppresses the induction of connective tissue growth factor by transforming growth factor-beta in normal and scleroderma fibroblasts. J Biol Chem 2000;275:15220–5.

[52] Mori R, Kondo T, Ohshima T, et al. Accelerated wound healing in tumor necrosis factor receptor p55-deficient mice with reduced leukocyte infiltration. FASEB J 2002;16:963–74.

[53] Boehm U, Klamp T, Groot M, et al. Cellular responses to interferon-gamma. Annu Rev Immunol 1997;15:749–95.

[54] Murayama Y, Vinuela F, Suzuki Y, et al. Ion implantation and protein coating of detachable coils for endovascular treatment of cerebral aneurysms: concepts and preliminary results in swine models. Neurosurgery 1997;40:1233–43; discussion, 1243–4.

[55] Murayama Y, Vinuela F, Suzuki Y, et al. Development of the biologically active Guglielmi detachable coil for the treatment of cerebral aneurysms. Part II: an experimental study in a swine aneurysm model. AJNR Am J Neuroradiol 1999;20:1992–9.

[56] Kallmes DF, Fujiwara NH, Yuen D, et al. A collagen-based coil for embolization of saccular aneurysms in a New Zealand White rabbit model. AJNR Am J Neuroradiol 2003;24:591–6.

[57] de Gast AN, Altes TA, Marx WF, et al. Transforming growth factor beta-coated platinum coils for endovascular treatment of aneurysms: an animal study. Neurosurgery 2001;49:690–4; discussion, 694–6.

[58] Desfaits AC, Raymond J, Muizelaar JP. Growth factors stimulate neointimal cells in vitro and increase the thickness of the neointima formed at the neck of porcine aneurysms treated by embolization. Stroke 2000;31:498–507.

[59] Venne D, Raymond J, Allas S, et al. Healing of experimental aneurysms. II: Platelet extracts can increase the thickness of the neointima at the neck of treated aneurysms. J Neuroradiol 1999;26: 92–100.

[60] Chen CH, Poucher SM, Lu J, et al. Fibroblast growth factor 2: from laboratory evidence to clinical application. Curr Vasc Pharmacol 2004;2:33–43.

[61] Hatano T, Miyamoto S, Kawakami O, et al. Acceleration of aneurysm healing by controlled release of basic fibroblast growth factor with the use of polyethylene terephthalate fiber coils coated with gelatin hydrogel. Neurosurgery 2003;53:393–400; discussion, 400–1.

[62] Kallmes DF, Williams AD, Cloft HJ, et al. Platinum coil-mediated implantation of growth factor-secreting endovascular tissue grafts: an in vivo study. Radiology 1998;207:519–23.

[63] Marx WE, Cloft HJ, Helm GA, et al. Endovascular treatment of experimental aneurysms by use of biologically modified embolic devices: coil-mediated intraaneurysmal delivery of fibroblast tissue allografts. AJNR Am J Neuroradiol 2001;22:323–33.

[64] Athanasiou KA, Agrawal CM, Barber FA, et al. Orthopaedic applications for PLA-PGA biodegradable polymers. Arthroscopy 1998;14:726–37.

[65] Atala A. Tissue engineering in urology. Curr Urol Rep 2001;2:83–92.

[66] Webb AR, Yang J, Ameer GA. Biodegradable polyester elastomers in tissue engineering. Expert Opin Biol Ther 2004;4:801–12.

[67] Salthouse TN. Biologic response to sutures. Otolaryngol Head Neck Surg 1980;88:658–64.

[68] Craig PH, Williams JA, Davis KW, et al. A biologic comparison of polyglactin 910 and polyglycolic acid synthetic absorbable sutures. Surg Gynecol Obstet 1975;141:1–10.

[69] Miller RA, Brady JM, Cutright DE. Degradation rates of oral resorbable implants (polylactates and polyglycolates): rate modification with changes in PLA/PGA copolymer ratios. J Biomed Mater Res 1977;11:711–9.

[70] Murayama Y, Vinuela F, Tateshima S, et al. Cellular responses of bioabsorbable polymeric material and Guglielmi detachable coil in experimental aneurysms. Stroke 2002;33:1120–8.

[71] Murayama Y, Tateshima S, Gonzalez NR, et al. Matrix and bioabsorbable polymeric coils accelerate healing of intracranial aneurysms: long-term experimental study. Stroke 2003;34:2031–7.

[72] Murayama Y, Vinuela F, Tateshima S, et al. Bioabsorbable polymeric material coils for embolization of intracranial aneurysms: a preliminary experimental study. J Neurosurg 2001;94:454–63.

[73] Kallmes DF, Fujiwara NH. New expandable hydrogel-platinum coil hybrid device for aneurysm embolization. AJNR Am J Neuroradiol 2002;23:1580–8.

[74] Cloft HJ, Kallmes DF. Aneurysm packing with HydroCoil Embolic System versus platinum coils: initial clinical experience. AJNR Am J Neuroradiol 2004;25:60–2.

ELSEVIER
SAUNDERS

Neurosurg Clin N Am 16 (2005) 501–516

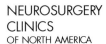

NEUROSURGERY
CLINICS
OF NORTH AMERICA

Endovascular Treatment of Cerebral Vasospasm: Transluminal Balloon Angioplasty, Intra-Arterial Papaverine, and Intra-Arterial Nicardipine

Brian L. Hoh, MD[a,b,*], Christopher S. Ogilvy, MD[b]

[a]Endovascular Neurosurgery, Neurosurgical Service, Massachusetts General Hospital,
Harvard Medical School, VBK 710, 55 Fruit Street, Boston, MA 02114, USA
[b]Cerebrovascular Surgery, Neurosurgical Service, Massachusetts General Hospital,
Harvard Medical School, VBK 710, 55 Fruit Street, Boston, MA 02114, USA

Cerebral vasospasm remains one of the leading causes of morbidity and mortality with subarachnoid hemorrhage [1], and it is seen angiographically in 70% and clinically in 20% to 30% of patients with aneurysmal subarachnoid hemorrhage [2,3]. In a study of serial CT scans in 619 consecutive patients with subarachnoid hemorrhage treated at the Massachusetts General Hospital, vasospasm was the leading cause for new infarcts in patients treated with surgical clipping or endovascular coiling [4].

A number of reports contend that there is lower incidence of cerebral vasospasm in patients with aneurysmal subarachnoid hemorrhage treated with endovascular coiling compared with surgical clipping [5–8]. We studied 515 consecutive patients with subarachnoid hemorrhage treated at the Massachusetts General Hospital using multivariate statistical methods controlling for clinical and radiologic factors, such as patient age, neurologic condition (Hunt and Hess grade), amount of hemorrhage on the CT scan (Fisher score), and aneurysm location, and found no difference in the incidence of vasospasm between endovascular coiling and surgical clipping [9]. In the patients treated with surgical clipping, there was 63% vasospasm, of which 28% was symptomatic. In the patients treated with endovascular coiling, there was 54% vasospasm, of which 33% was symptomatic (no statistical difference) [9].

Significant hemorrhage on the CT scan (Fisher score of 3 or 4) and poor neurologic condition (Hunt and Hess grade of 4 or 5) significantly predicted symptomatic vasospasm, and symptomatic vasospasm was a strong predictor of poor clinical outcome and in-hospital mortality [9].

Transluminal balloon angioplasty

Although medical management of cerebral vasospasm consists largely of nimodipine and hypertensive hyperdynamic therapy [10], there are patients who experience vasospasm refractory to these therapies. Endovascular treatment can be effective in these patients with medically refractory vasospasm.

In 1984, Zubkov and colleagues [11] were the first to report using a balloon catheter for angioplasty of cerebral vessels in vasospasm. Since then, there have been a number of clinical studies reporting series of patients with cerebral vasospasm treated with transluminal balloon angioplasty [12–29] (Table 1; Fig. 1). The efficacy of transluminal balloon angioplasty to reverse neurologic deficits related to cerebral vasospasm is variably reported in the literature as ranging from 11% to 93%. We reviewed the literature to date in the English language for reports of clinical series of endovascular therapy for cerebral vasospasm, and from selected reports, there were 530 patients treated with transluminal balloon angioplasty for cerebral vasospasm, of whom 328 (62%) improved clinically (see Table 1).

* Corresponding author.
E-mail address: bhoh@partners.org (B.L. Hoh).

Table 1
Selected series of transluminal balloon angioplasty for cerebral vasospasm in the literature

Authors	Number of patients	Clinical improvement	Transcranial doppler	Cerebral blood flow	Major complications	Vessel rupture
Newell et al [12]	10	8/10 patients (80%) improved	2/2 patients (100%) improved		3/10 patients (30%)	0/10 patients (0%)
Higashida et al [13]	13	10/13 patients (77%) improved or remained in excellent condition			1/13 patients (7.7%)	0/13 patients (0%)
Newell et al [14]	41	28/39 patients (72%) improved, 2 performed prophylactically	27/29 patients (93%) improved	SPECT: 8/10 patients (80%) improved	4/41 patients (9.8%)	1/41 patients (2.4%)
Zubkov et al [15]	95	82/95 patients (87%) improved		^{133}Xe-clearance: 62/69 patients (90%) improved [16]	4/95 patients (4.5%)	1/95 patients (1%)
Mayberg et al [17]; Eskridge et al [18]	50	32/50 patients (64%) improved	"In patients demonstrating clinical improvement, TCD blood flow velocities decreased and remained below pre-angioplasty levels." [17]	"Improvement in cerebral perfusion was demonstrated by resolution of perfusion defects on SPECT scans in the majority of patients." [17]	5/50 patients (10%)	1/50 patients (2%)
Coyne et al [19]	13	4/13 patients (31%) improved			1/13 patients (8%)	0/13 patients (0%)
Fujii et al [20]	19	12/19 patients (63%) improved		SPECT: 3/5 patients (60%) improved		
Takis et al [21]	8	5/8 patients (63%) good outcome			1/8 patients (12.5%)	0/8 patients (0%)
Terada et al [22]	7	5/7 patients (71%) GOS 1-2 outcomes			0/7 patients (0%)	0/7 patients (0%)
Firlik et al [23]	13	12/13 patients (93%) improved		^{133}Xe-CT: 12/12 patients (100%) improved mean CBF in at-risk regions of interest. Pre-TBA to post-TBA mean CBF: 13 ± 2.1 to 44 ± 13.1 ml/100g/min ($P < 0.00005$)	1/13 patients (7.7%)	0/13 patients (0%)

Study	N	Outcome	Velocities	Imaging	Complications	Mortality
Elliot et al [24]	39	30/39 patients (77%) improved	Pre-TBA to post-TBA mean velocity: 166 ± 9 to 92 ± 4 cm/sec (P < 0.001)	SPECT: 30/42 territories (71%) improved	1/39 patients (2.5%)	0/39 patients (0%)
Bejjani et al [25]	31	22/31 patients (72%) improved			3/31 patients (9.7%)	0/31 patients (0%)
Rosenwasser et al [32]	93	36/93 patients (39%) good outcomes at >6 months			0/93 patients (0%)	0/93 patients (0%)
Muizelaar et al [26]	13 prophylactic	no patient developed DIND, 10/13 patients (77%) favorable outcome	no velocities >200 cm/sec		1/13 patients (7.7%)	1/13 patients (7.7%)
Polin et al [27]	38	4/38 patients (11%) immediate improvement; 11/38 patients (29%) improvement at 4 day follow-up	15/38 patients (39%) patients improved		"In our series, it was impossible to determine if any of the unfavorable outcomes were caused by complications of vasospasm."	
Oskouian et al [28]	12	6/12 patients (50%) improved	Decreased mean velocities post-TBA: MCA 12/12 patients (100%) EC-ICA 10/12 patients (84%) hemispheric ratio 10/12 patients (84%) MCA spasm index 12/12 patients (100%) Pre-TBA to post-TBA mean velocities: MCA 157.6 ± 9.4 to 76.3 ± 9.3 cm/sec (P < 0.05) EC-ICA 31.0±3.7 to 39.9±3.8 cm/sec (P = NS) hemispheric ratio 4.1 ± 2.9 to 2.5 ± 3.0 cm/sec (P = NS) MCA spasm index 6.1 ± 0.4 to 2.8 ± 0.5 cm/sec (P < 0.05)	^{133}Xe-clearance: 7/12 patients (58%) improved. Pre-TBA to post-TBA mean CBF: 27.8±2.8 to 28.4 ± 3.0 ml/100g/min (P = NS)	0/12 patients (0%)	

(continued on next page)

Table 1 (continued)

Authors	Number of patients	Clinical improvement	Transcranial doppler	Cerebral blood flow	Major complications	Vessel rupture
Rabinstein et al [29]	35	15/35 patients (43%) good outcomes			2/105 procedures (TBA and/or IAP) (1.9%)	1/35 patients (2.9%)
Total	530	328/530 patients (62%) with improvement or good outcome	56/81 patients (69%) improved	92/108 patients (85%) improved; 30/42 territories (71%) improved	27/543 patients or procedures (5.0%)	5/473 patients (1.1%)

Abbreviations: CBF, cerebral blood flow; DIND, delayed ischemic neurologic deficit; EC-ICA, exracranial-internal carotid artery; MCA, middle cerebral artery; NS, not significant; SPECT, serial single photon emission computerized tomography; TBA, transluminal balloon angioplasty; TCD, transcranial doppler ultrasonography; Xe, xenon.

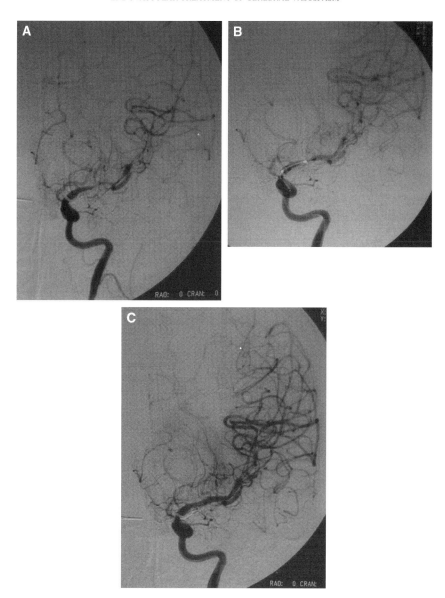

Fig. 1. Transluminal balloon angioplasty for cerebral vasospasm. (*A*) AP left internal carotid artery (ICA) injection digital subtraction angiography (DSA) demonstrating severe vasospasm of the left middle cerebral artery (MCA). (*B*) Transluminal balloon angioplasty of the left MCA. (*C*) Post-angioplasty AP left ICA injection DSA demonstrating angiographic reversal of vasospasm in the left MCA.

Transluminal balloon angioplasty is not without its complications, however. Complications can include arterial dissection, thromboembolism, branch occlusion [14,27], reperfusion hemorrhage into infarcted territories [13], bleeding from unsecured aneurysms [14,27], and vessel rupture [14,15,17,18,26,29–31]. In our review of selected reports in the English language literature in which complications were reported of transluminal balloon angioplasty, there were major complications in 5.0% and vessel rupture occurred in 1.1% (see Table 1).

Several reports have demonstrated improvement in transcranial Doppler (TCD) ultrasonography flow velocities after compared with before transluminal balloon angioplasty. There are two methods in which this has been reported: to report the number of patients in whom TCD velocities improved or to report the mean TCD velocities for the cohort of patients after compared with before transluminal balloon angioplasty. Using the former method, several studies have demonstrated that TCD velocities were improved after compared with before transluminal balloon angioplasty in 39% to 100% of patients [12,14,27,28]. In our review of selected reports in the English language literature, of 81 patients in whom before and after transluminal balloon angioplasty TCD velocities were reported, there were 56 (69%) in whom TCD velocities improved (see Table 1). The latter method of reporting TCD velocities has been reported in several studies as well. Elliott and coworkers [24] demonstrated improvement in mean TCD velocities from 166 ± 9 cm/s before transluminal balloon angioplasty to 92 ± 4 cm/s after transluminal balloon angioplasty ($P < 0.001$). Oskouian and colleagues [28] reported improvement in mean TCD velocities before and after transluminal balloon angioplasty of the middle cerebral artery (MCA) and external carotid artery (ECA)–internal carotid artery (ICA) as well as in hemispheric ratios and the MCA spasm index: 157.6 ± 9.4 to 76.3 ± 9.3 cm/s ($P < .05$), 31.0 ± 3.7 to 39.9 ± 3.8 cm/s ($P =$ not significant), 4.1 ± 2.9 to 2.5 ± 3.0 cm/s ($P =$ not significant), and 6.1 ± 0.4 to 2.8 ± 0.5 cm/s ($P < .05$), respectively.

The effect of transluminal balloon angioplasty on cerebral blood flow (CBF) has been demonstrated with perfusion techniques: ^{133}Xenon clearance, ^{133}Xenon CT, or serial single photon emission computerized tomography (SPECT). Using ^{133}Xenon clearance techniques, a few reports have demonstrated improvement in CBF in 58% to 90% of patients treated with transluminal balloon angioplasty [16,28]. When the mean CBF for the cohort in one study was compared before and after transluminal balloon angioplasty, however, there was not a statistical difference before (27.8 ± 2.8 mL/100 g/min) compared with after (28.4 ± 3.0 mL/100 g/min) ($P =$ not significant) [28]. Firlik and coworkers [23] used ^{133}Xenon CT and demonstrated that all 12 patients (100%) they studied had an improved mean CBF in at-risk regions of interest (ROIs). They also reported a significant improvement in before to after transluminal balloon angioplasty mean CBF: 13 ± 2.1 mL/100 g/min to 44 ± 13.1 mL/100 g/min ($P < .00005$) [23]. Other studies used SPECT to demonstrate improvement in CBF in 60% to 80% of patients [14,20] or an improvement in CBF to 71% of territories treated [24]. In our review of

selected reports in the English language literature, of 108 patients in whom before and after transluminal balloon angioplasty CBF was studied by perfusion techniques, there were 92 patients (85%) in whom CBF improved (see Table 1).

The optimal timing of transluminal balloon angioplasty in relation to the onset of cerebral vasospasm or signs and symptoms is not well defined. Rosenwasser and colleagues [32] reported significantly better and sustained clinical outcomes in patients they had treated with transluminal balloon angioplasty within 2 hours of symptom onset (70% improvement) compared with patients they had treated at more than 2 hours after symptom onset (40% improvement) in a retrospective non–case-controlled review of the patients' outcomes. Muizelaar and coworkers [26] performed a pilot study of prophylactic transluminal balloon angioplasty for patients with Fisher grade 3 subarachnoid hemorrhage. Of the 13 patients reported in the pilot study, no patient developed delayed ischemic neurologic deficit and 10 (77%) of the 13 patients had favorable outcomes. TCD ultrasonography was performed, and none of the 13 patients had postangioplasty TCD velocities greater than 200 cm/s. There was, however, 1 patient who died after vessel rupture during transluminal balloon angioplasty, resulting in a complication rate of 7.7%.

Although the exact mechanisms for the effects of transluminal balloon angioplasty are not entirely elucidated, there have been several animal and human autopsy studies to examine this question. In a study of nonhuman primates (*Macaca fuscata* monkeys), scanning electron microscopy and transmission electron microscopy demonstrated that untreated vessels in vasospasm were characterized by endothelial convolutions and marked corrugations of the internal elastic lamina, whereas vessels treated with angioplasty were characterized by flatter convolutions, the corrugated internal elastic lamina was extended, and there was only slight endothelial cell damage [33]. In a study in which scanning electron microscopy was performed in three patients at autopsy of vessels with vasospasm that were treated with angioplasty compared with vessels with vasospasm that were untreated, the untreated vessels in vasospasm demonstrated proliferation of connective tissue in the media and intima, whereas vessels treated with angioplasty demonstrated thinning of the arterial wall by compression and stretching, without disruption of cellular and connective tissue elements and without damage to the endothelium [34]. Several other human autopsy and animal studies have demonstrated the same mechanism for the effects of transluminal balloon angioplasty, that is, compression of the connective tissue which proliferates in the setting of cerebral vasospasm, stretching of the internal elastic lamina, and a combination of compression and stretching of the smooth muscle [35–37].

Intra-arterial papaverine

With the early successful results reported with transluminal balloon angioplasty, there was enthusiasm for developing vasodilating agents that could be delivered intra-arterially as an endovascular therapy for medically refractory vasospasm. Not only were there associated risks of complications with transluminal balloon angioplasty, but navigation of balloon catheters has been limited primarily to the proximal cerebral vessels. Thus, there was hope that intra-arterial injection of vasodilating agents could theoretically treat vasospasm of distal cerebral vessels [38]. Papaverine hydrochloride is a benzylisoquinoline alkaloid derivative of opium known to cause arterial dilatation, probably from inhibition of arterial smooth muscle contraction by phosphodiesterase inhibition. In 1992, Kaku and colleagues [39] were the first to report the intra-arterial injection of papaverine to treat cerebral vasospasm. Since then, there have been a number of clinical series reporting variable results and associated complications with intra-arterial papaverine therapy [24,28,29,39–53] (Table 2). The efficacy of intra-arterial papaverine to improve clinical outcomes in patients with cerebral vasospasm is variably reported in the literature, ranging from 0% to 100%. We reviewed the literature to date in the English language for clinical series of intra-arterial papaverine therapy for cerebral vasospasm, and from selected reports, there were 346 patients treated with intra-arterial papaverine therapy for cerebral vasospasm, of whom 148 (43%) improved clinically (see Table 2).

A significant criticism of intra-arterial papaverine therapy is the relatively short duration of its beneficial effects and the recurrence of vasospasm after treatment. Patients with severe cerebral vasospasm often require more than one session of intra-arterial papaverine treatment. In 2004, Liu and coworkers [53] reported on 17 patients who underwent 91 total sessions of multiple intra-arterial papaverine treatment (5.4 sessions per patient). In our review of selected reports from the English language literature, there were 401 patients who underwent 663 treatment sessions of intra-arterial papaverine, for a mean of 1.7 treatment sessions per patient (see Table 2). Papaverine's effect on vessels has a relatively short half-life. Milburn and colleagues [38] reported excellent angiographic results in patients treated with intra-arterial papaverine therapy, as demonstrated by their measurement of vessel diameters in proximal and distal vessels; however, 9 of the patients underwent repeat angiography the next day, and all had recurrent arterial narrowing. Elliott and colleagues [24] reported that the beneficial effect of intra-arterial papaverine on TCD velocities did not last up to 48 hours. Vajkoczy and colleagues [51] reported that improvement of CBF after intra-arterial papaverine treatment did not continue for up to 12 hours after treatment. Another explanation may be the concept that vessels in vasospasm may be initially responsive to papaverine within a certain time window after subarachnoid hemorrhage but that after an interval of time, they become resistant to papaverine because of histologic changes that have occurred in the vessels or because of a cascade of pathophysiologic events that have taken place. This vessel-responsive phase theory of papaverine's effects in cerebral vasospasm has been demonstrated in a number of animal studies [54–57].

The effect of intra-arterial papaverine on TCD velocities has been reported. Variable results have been reported, ranging from 39% to 85% of patients treated with intra-arterial papaverine therapy reported as having had improvement in their TCD velocities after treatment [28,47]. Other reports have demonstrated significant improvement in mean TCD velocities comparing before and after treatment for cohorts of patients who underwent intra-arterial papaverine therapy. In our review of selected reports in the English language literature, of 51 patients in whom before and after intra-arterial papaverine TCD velocities were reported, there were 29 patients (57%) in whom TCD velocities improved (see Table 2). Yoshimura and colleagues [44] reported improvement in before to after intra-arterial papaverine treatment mean TCD velocities from 100.9 ± 18.6 cm/s to 59.0 ± 18 cm/s ($P < .01$). Likewise, Vajkoczy and coworkers [51] reported improvement in mean TCD velocities in the MCA from 207.3 ± 22.0 cm/s to 152.2 ± 25.3 cm/s ($P < .05$). Oskouian and colleagues [28] reported significant improvements in mean TCD velocities for

Table 2
Selected series of Intra-arterial Papaverine (IAP) therapy for cerebral vasospasm in the literature

Authors	Number of patients	Number of territories	Number of treatments	Clinical improvement	Transcranial doppler	Cerebral blood flow	Complications	Total complications
Kaku et al [39]	10	37	10 (1.0/pt)	8/10 patients (80%) improved			0/10 patients (0%)	0/10 patients (0%)
Kassell et al [40]	12	16	14 (1.2/pt)	4/12 patients (33%) improved			1/12 transient hemiparesis and mental status change (8.3%) 1/12 pupillary dilation (8.3%)	2/12 patients (17%)
Marks et al [41]	2	4	4 (2.0/pt)	1/2 patients (50%) improved			1/2 seizures (50%)	1/2 seizures (50%)
Clouston et al [42]	14	60	19 (1.4/pt)	7/14 patients (50%) improved			1/14 monocular blindness (7.1%) 1/14 arterial dissection (7.1%) 1/14 seizure (7.1%)	3/14 patients (21%)
McAuliffe et al [43]	21	42	27 (1.3/pt)	11/21 patients (52%) improved			1/21 fatal vessel rupture (4.8%) 1/21 large infarct, epidural hematoma (4.8%) 1/21 fatal basal ganglia hemorrhage (4.8%)	3/21 patients (14%)
Yoshimura et al [44]	19	19	19 (1.0/pt)	15/19 patients (79%) improved	Pre-IAP to Post-IAP mean velocity: 100.9 ± 18.6 to 59.0 ± 18 cm/sec ($P < 0.01$)		0/19 patients (0%)	0/19 patients (0%)
Sawada et al [45]	46	90	46 (1.0/pt)	11/46 patients (24%) improved			4/46 transient plegia/paresis (8.7%) 4/46 pupillary dilation (8.7%) 1/46 transient mental status changes (2.2%)	9/46 patients (20%)
Cross et al [46]	28	78	51 (1.8/pt)	not reported			1/28 arrest (3.6%) 1/28 seizure (3.6%) 2/28 transient aphasia (7.1%) 3/28 mental status changes (11%)	7/28 patients (25%)

Polin et al [47]	31	not reported	46 (1.5/pt)	4/31 patients (13%) immediate improvement; 12/31 patients (39%) improvement at 4 day F/U	12/31 patients (39%) improved	not reported	not reported	not reported
Fandino et al [48]	10	23	10 (1.0/pt)	10/10 patients (100%) improved		SVJO2: 9/10 patients (90%) improved; Pre-IAP to post-IAP means SVJO2 improved ($P < 0.01$)	0/10 patients (0%)	0/10 patients (0%)
Elliott et al [24]	13	24	21 (1.6/pt)	9/13 patients (69%) improved with initial treatment	Pre-IAP to post-IAP mean velocity: 158 ± 8 to 127 ± 13 cm/sec ($P < 0.01$) mean MCA velocity: 166 ± 10 to 135 ± 15 cm/sec ($P < 0.05$) IC/EC ratio: 4.1 ± 0.4 to 3.7 ± 0.5 ($P = NS$) *all changes were only transient and did not maintain to post-treatment day 2	SPECT: 5/16 territories (31%) improved	0/13 patients (0%)	0/13 patients (0%)
Firlik et al [49]	15	32	23 (1.5/pt)	6/23 treatments (26%)		^{133}Xe-CT: 6/13 patients (46%) had reduction in number of at-risk regions of interest	1/23 worsened vasospasm, hemispheric infarction (4.3%) 1/23 transient brainstem depression (4.3%) 1/23 seizure (4.3%) 1/23 profound hypotension (4.3%)	4/23 treatments (17%) [3/15 patients (20%)]
Zervas and Ogilvy [50]	39	142	91 (2.3/pt)	not reported			6/39 arterial dissections (15%) 13/39 embolic infarcts (33%)	19/39 patients (49%)

(continued on next page)

Table 2 (continued)

Authors	Number of patients	Number of territories	Number of treatments	Clinical improvement	Transcranial doppler	Cerebral blood flow	Complications	Total complications
Vajkoczy et al [51]	8	10	8 (1.0/pt)	0/12 patients (0%) good outcomes	Pre-IAP to post-IAP mean MCA velocity: 207.3 ± 22.0 to 152.2 ± 25.3 cm/sec (P < 0.05)	Thermal dilution: Pre-IAP to post IAP: 7.3 ± 1.6 to 37.9 ± 6.6 ml/100 gm/min (P < 0.05) only transient, did not maintain for long-term (up to 12 hours)	not reported	not reported
Andaluz et al [52]	50	166	94 (1.88/pt)	13/50 patients (26%)			5/50 fatal sustained increased ICP (10%) 1/50 transient aphasia and hemiplegia (2.0%) 1/50 pupillary dilation (2.0%) 1/50 brainstem depression (2.0%) 1/50 aneurysm perforation (2.0%)	9/50 patients (18%)
Oskouian et al [28]	20	not reported	24 (1.2/pt)	9/20 patients (45%) improved	Decreased mean velocities post-IAP: MCA 17/20 patients (85%) EC-ICA 7/20 patients (35%) hemispheric ratio 8/20 patients (40%) MCA spasm index 14/20 patients (70%) Pre-IAP to post-IAP mean velocities: MCA 109.9 ± 9.1 to 82.8 ± 8.6 cm/sec (P < 0.05) EC-ICA 33.1 ± 3.6 to 35.2 ± 3.4 cm/sec (P = NS) hemispheric ratio 3.3 ± 2.9 to 2.8 ± 0.3 cm/sec (P = NS) MCA spasm index 4.4 ± 0.3 to 2.5 ± 0.3 cm/sec (P < 0.05)	^{133}133Xe-clearance: 11/20 patients (55%) improved Pre-IAP to post-IAP mean CBF: 27.5 ± 2.1 to 38.7 ± 2.8 ml/100 g/min (P < 0.05)	0/20 patients (0%)	0/20 patients (0%)

Liu et al [53]	17	33	91 (5.4/pt)	12/17 patients (71%) improved	29/51 patients (57%) improved	1/17 transient aphasia (5.9%)	1/17 patients (5.9%)
Rabinstein et al [29]	46	not reported	65 (1.4/pt)	20/46 patients (43%) good outcomes	26/43 patients (60%) improved; 5/16 territories (31%) improved	2/105 treatments (TBA and/or IAP) (1.9%)	2/105 treatments (TBA and/or IAP) (1.9%)
Total	401	>873*	663 (1.7/pt)	148/346 patients (43%) with improvement or good outcome			60/609 treatments (9.9%)

Abbreviations: CBF, cerebral blood flow; IAP, intra-arterial papaverine; IC/EC, intracranial to extracranial; ICP, intracranial pressure; MCA, middle cerebral artery; NS, not significant; SPECT, serial single photon emission computerized tomography; SVJO2, jugular venous bulb oxygen saturation; TCD, transcranial doppler ultrasonography; Xe, xenon.

* Some series did not report the number of vascular territories treated. In those instances, it was assumed that at least one territory was treated for each patient. Therefore, there was at least 873 territories altogether.

the MCA (109.9 ± 9.1 cm/s to 82.8 ± 8.6 cm/s; $P < .05$) and in the MCA spasm index (4.4 ± 0.3 cm/s to 2.5 ± 0.3 cm/s; $P < .05$), but non-significant differences for the ECA-ICA ratios and hemispheric ratios. Finally, Elliott and coworkers [24] reported significant improvements in overall mean TCD velocities (158 ± 8 cm/s to 127 ± 13 cm/s; $P < .01$) and mean TCD MCA velocities (166 ± 10 cm/s to 135 ± 15 cm/s; $P < .05$); however, these improvements were only transient and did not continue to 2 days after intra-arterial papaverine treatment.

Intra-arterial papaverine's effect on CBF has been studied with thermal dilution techniques, jugular venous bulb oxygen saturation, ^{133}Xenon clearance, ^{133}Xenon CT, and serial SPECT. Fandino and colleagues [48] studied jugular venous bulb oxygen saturation to demonstrate significant improvement in CBF in 9 of 10 patients with cerebral vasospasm after intra-arterial papaverine treatment and reported a significant improvement in the overall mean jugular venous bulb oxygen saturation ($P < .01$). Elliott and coworkers [24] used SPECT techniques to demonstrate improvement in CBF in 5 (31%) of 16 vascular territories studied. Vajkoczy and colleagues [51] used thermal dilution techniques to demonstrate improvement from before to after intra-arterial papaverine treatment CBF of 7.3 ± 1.6 mL/100 g/min to 37.9 ± 6.6 mL/100 gm/min ($P < .05$); however, this improvement was only transient and did not continue for up to 12 hours after treatment. Firlik and coworkers [49] studied ^{133}Xenon CT and reported that 6 (46%) of 13 patients had a reduction in the number of at-risk ROIs in CBF. Oskouian and colleagues [28] used ^{133}Xenon clearance to demonstrate significant improvement in CBF after intra-arterial papaverine treatment in 11 (55%) of 20 patients and improvement in mean CBF from before to after intra-arterial papaverine treatment of 27.5 ± 2.1 mL/100 g/min to 38.7 ± 2.8 mL/100 g/min ($P < .05$). In our review of selected reports in the English language literature, of 43 patients in whom before and after intra-arterial papaverine CBF was studied by perfusion techniques, there were 26 patients (60%) in whom CBF improved and 5 (31%) of 16 vascular territories that improved (see Table 2).

One of the most important limitations of intra-arterial papaverine therapy is its effect of increasing intracranial pressure (ICP) [43,46,52]. Cross and colleagues [46] demonstrated that ICP increases with intra-arterial papaverine therapy were significantly associated with adverse outcomes, and

Andaluz and colleagues [52] reported a 10% mortality rate from papaverine-induced ICP. The ICP elevations seem to be related to the rate of papaverine administration [46]. The mechanism of increased ICP associated with intra-arterial papaverine is not known; however, it has been speculated that it may have to do with the non-selective dilatation effects of papaverine, resulting in vasodilation and increased capacitance in the venous bed [46,52]. It is strongly cautioned that any intra-arterial papaverine therapy be performed with continuous ICP monitoring [43,46,52].

In the 1990s at the Massachusetts General Hospital, intra-arterial papaverine therapy was used to treat medical refractory vasospasm. We encountered a significant number of complications, however, as we reported previously [50]. In 39 patients in whom 142 vessels were treated with 91 treatment sessions of intra-arterial papaverine, there were 6 arterial dissections (15%) and 13 embolic infarcts (33%) [50]. Papaverine treatment for cerebral vasospasm has also been associated with seizures, the mechanism of which is unknown [22,41,42,46,49,58–60], monocular blindness [42], brain stem dysfunction [49,52,61,62], neurologic deficits that resolve after stopping papaverine infusion [39,40,45,46,52,53], hemorrhage [43], pupillary dilation [40,45,52], respiratory arrest [46], profound hypotension [49], aneurysm perforation [52], formation of crystal precipitate emboli [63], and even paradoxic worsening of vasospasm [49,64]. In our review of selected reports in the English language literature, of 609 treatment sessions with intra-arterial papaverine therapy, there were 60 complications (9.9%) (see Table 2).

Smith and colleagues [65] reported neurotoxic effects of intra-arterial papaverine. In five patients who exhibited neurologic deterioration with papaverine treatment, they demonstrated selective gray matter only signal changes within the territories infused with papaverine on MRI. Histologic analysis performed on autopsy of one of the patients demonstrated selective injury to islands of neurons with relative sparing of white matter [65].

Elliott and colleagues [24] directly compared transluminal balloon angioplasty and intra-arterial papaverine therapy for treatment of cerebral vasospasm. They found transluminal balloon angioplasty to be superior to intra-arterial papaverine because of greater sustained improvements in TCD velocities, greater improvement in cerebral perfusion as demonstrated by SPECT scanning, and fewer treatment failures. Transluminal balloon angioplasty resulted in permanent reversal of

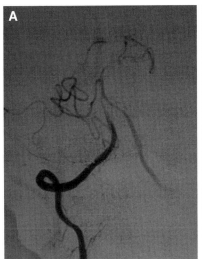
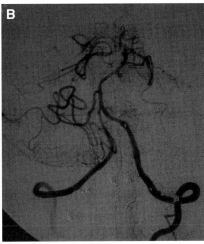

Fig. 2. Intra-arterial nicardipine infusion for cerebral vasospasm. (*A*) AP right vertebral artery (VA) injection digital subtraction angiography (DSA) demonstrating severe vasospasm of the vertebrobasilar system. (*B*) Post-intra-arterial nicardipine AP left VA injection DSA demonstrating angiographic reversal of vasospasm in the vertebrobasilar system.

vasospasm in the cerebral vessels, whereas patients treated with intra-arterial papaverine often required retreatment [24].

Intra-arterial nicardipine

For a number of reasons, including the significant number of complications we encountered using intra-arterial papaverine at the Massachusetts General Hospital in the 1990s [50], the lack of sustained treatment effect of papaverine, the need for multiple treatments, and the associated increases in ICP [43,46,52], we have abandoned using papaverine and have used nicardipine as our intra-arterial vasodilating agent for the endovascular treatment of cerebral vasospasm (Fig. 2).

Nicardipine is a dihydropyridine calcium antagonist with an apparent selective dilatation effect on vascular smooth muscle over cardiac muscle. Initially, it was studied as an intravenous agent for prophylactic treatment against the development of cerebral vasospasm and was shown to have beneficial effects in lowering the incidence of angiographic and clinical vasospasm [66–69].

We have previously reported our initial experience with intra-arterial nicardipine therapy for cerebral vasospasm at the Massachusetts General Hospital [70]. In a 12-month span, we treated 48 vessels in 24 patients with intra-arterial nicardipine alone or in addition to transluminal balloon angioplasty. We reported on 18 patients who underwent only intra-arterial nicardipine treatment in 44 vessels. There was angiographic and TCD improvement in all cases. Clinical improvement occurred in 8 patients (42%). Mean TCD velocities were significantly improved before to after intra-arterial nicardipine treatment from 268.9 ± 77.8 cm/s to 197.6 ± 74.1 cm/s ($P < .001$) and were sustained for 4 days after treatment. The only adverse effect occurred in 1 patient in whom there was an increase in ICP, which necessitated termination of the intra-arterial nicardipine infusion. There were no hemodynamic changes with nicardipine infusion.

Based on this experience, we have adopted a current treatment protocol of transluminal balloon angioplasty or intra-arterial nicardipine therapy as endovascular treatment for medically refractory cerebral vasospasm.

References

[1] Kassell NF, Torner JC, Haley EC Jr, et al. The International Cooperative Study on the Timing of Aneurysm Surgery. Part 1: overall management results. J Neurosurg 1990;73:18–36.
[2] Kassell NF, Sasaki T, Colohan ART, et al. Cerebral vasospasm following aneurysmal subarachnoid hemorrhage. Stroke 1985;16:562–72.

[3] Weir B, Macdonald RL, Stoodley M. Etiology of cerebral vasospasm. Acta Neurochir (Wien) 1999; 72:27–46.

[4] Hoh BL, Curry WT Jr, Carter BS, et al. Computed tomographic demonstrated infarcts after surgical and endovascular treatment of aneurysmal subarachnoid hemorrhage. Acta Neurochir (Wien) 2004;146:1177–83.

[5] Rabinstein AA, Pichelmann MA, Friedman JA, et al. Symptomatic vasospasm and outcomes following aneurysmal subarachnoid hemorrhage: a comparison between surgical repair and endovascular coil occlusion. J Neurosurg 2003;98:319–25.

[6] Hohlrieder M, Spiegel M, Hinterhoelzl J, et al. Cerebral vasospasm and ischaemic infarction in clipped and coiled intracranial aneurysm patients. Eur J Neurol 2002;9:389–99.

[7] Murayama Y, Malisch T, Guglielmi G, et al. Incidence of cerebral vasospasm after endovascular treatment of acutely ruptured aneurysms: report on 69 cases. J Neurosurg 1997;87:830–5.

[8] Yalamanchili K, Rosenwasser RH, Thomas JE, et al. Frequency of cerebral vasospasm in patients treated with endovascular occlusion of intracranial aneurysms. AJNR Am J Neuroradiol 1998;19: 553–8.

[9] Hoh BL, Topcuoglu MA, Singhal AB, et al. Effect of clipping, craniotomy, or intravascular coiling on cerebral vasospasm and patient outcome after aneurysmal subarachnoid hemorrhage. Neurosurgery 2004;55:779–89.

[10] Hoh BL, Carter BS, Ogilvy CS. Risk of hemorrhage from unsecured, unruptured aneurysms during and after hypertensive hypervolemic therapy. Neurosurgery 2002;50:1207–11.

[11] Zubkov YN, Nikiforov BM, Shustin VA. Balloon catheter technique for dilatation of constricted cerebral arteries after aneurysmal SAH. Acta Neurochir (Wien) 1984;70:65–79.

[12] Newell DW, Eskridge JM, Mayberg MR, et al. Angioplasty for the treatment of symptomatic vasospasm following subarachnoid hemorrhage. J Neurosurg 1989;71:654–60.

[13] Higashida RT, Halbach VV, Cahan LD, et al. Transluminal angioplasty for treatment of intracranial arterial vasospasm. J Neurosurg 1989;71:648–53.

[14] Newell DW, Eskridge J, Mayberg M, et al. Endovascular treatment of intracranial aneurysms and cerebral vasospasm. Clin Neurosurg 1992;39: 348–60.

[15] Zubkov YN, Alexander LF, Benashvili GM, et al. Cerebral angioplasty for vasospasm. In: Findlay JM, editor. Cerebral vasospasm. Amsterdam: Elsevier Science Publishers BV; 1993. p. 321–4.

[16] Zubkov YN, Semenutin V, Benashvili GM, et al. Cerebral blood flow following angioplasty for vasospasm. In: Findlay JM, editor. Cerebral vasospasm. Amsterdam: Elsevier Science Publishers BV; 1993. p. 325–7.

[17] Mayberg M, Le Roux PD, Elliott JP, et al. Treatment of cerebral vasospasm with transluminal angioplasty. In: Findlay JM, editor. Cerebral vasospasm. Amsterdam: Elsevier Science Publishers BV; 1993. p. 329–32.

[18] Eskridge JM, McAuliffe W, Song JK, et al. Balloon angioplasty for the treatment of vasospasm: results of first 50 cases. Neurosurgery 1998;42: 510–6.

[19] Coyne TJ, Montanera WJ, MacDonald RL, et al. Transluminal angioplasty for cerebral vasospasm—the Toronto Hospital experience. In: Findlay JM, editor. Cerebral vasospasm. Amsterdam: Elsevier Science Publishers BV; 1993. p. 333–6.

[20] Fujii Y, Takahashi A, Yoshimoto T. Effect of balloon angioplasty on high grade symptomatic vasospasm after subarachnoid hemorrhage. Neurosurg Rev 1995;18:7–13.

[21] Takis C, Kwan ES, Pessin MS, et al. Intracranial angioplasty: experience and complications. AJNR Am J Neuroradiol 1997;18:1661–8.

[22] Terada T, Kinoshita Y, Yokote H, et al. The effect of endovascular therapy for cerebral arterial spasm, its limitation and pitfalls. Acta Neurochir (Wien) 1997; 139:227–34.

[23] Firlik AD, Kaufmann AM, Jungreis CA, et al. Effect of transluminal angioplasty on cerebral blood flow in the management of symptomatic vasospasm following aneurysmal subarachnoid hemorrhage. J Neurosurg 1997;86:830–9.

[24] Elliott JP, Newell DW, Lam DJ, et al. Comparison of balloon angioplasty and papaverine infusion for the treatment of vasospasm following aneurysmal subarachnoid hemorrhage. J Neurosurg 1998;88: 277–84.

[25] Bejjani GK, Bank WO, Olan WJ, et al. The efficacy and safety of angioplasty for cerebral vasospasm after subarachnoid hemorrhage. Neurosurgery 1998; 42:979–86.

[26] Muizelaar JP, Zwienenberg M, Rudisill NA, et al. The prophylactic use of transluminal balloon angioplasty in patients with Fisher Grade 3 subarachnoid hemorrhage: a pilot study. J Neurosurg 1999;91: 51–8.

[27] Polin RS, Coenen VA, Hansen CA, et al. Efficacy of transluminal angioplasty for the management of symptomatic cerebral vasospasm following aneurysmal subarachnoid hemorrhage. J Neurosurg 2000; 92:284–90.

[28] Oskouian RJ Jr, Martin NA, Lee JH, et al. Multimodal quantitation of the effects of endovascular therapy for vasospasm on cerebral blood flow, transcranial Doppler, ultrasonographic velocities, and cerebral artery diameters. Neurosurgery 2002;51: 30–43.

[29] Rabinstein AA, Friedman JA, Nichols DA, et al. Predictors of outcome after endovascular treatment of cerebral vasospasm. AJNR Am J Neuroradiol 2004;25:1778–82.

[30] Linskey ME, Horton JA, Rao GR, et al. Fatal rupture of the intracranial carotid artery during transluminal angioplasty for vasospasm induced by subarachnoid hemorrhage. Case report. J Neurosurg 1991;74:985–90.

[31] Volk EE, Prayson RA, Perl J II. Autopsy findings of fatal complication of posterior cerebral circulation angioplasty. Arch Pathol Lab Med 1997;121: 738–40.

[32] Rosenwasser RH, Armonda RA, Thomas JE, et al. Therapeutic modalities for the management of cerebral vasospasm: timing of endovascular options. Neurosurgery 1999;44:975–9.

[33] Kobayashi H, Ide H, Aradachi H, et al. Histological studies of intracranial vessels in primates following transluminal angioplasty for vasospasm. In: Findlay JM, editor. Cerebral vasospasm. Amsterdam: Elsevier Science Publishers BV; 1993. p. 345–8.

[34] Benashvili GM, Bernanke DH, Zubkov YN, et al. Angioplasty rearranges collagen after subarachnoid hemorrhage. In: Findlay JM, editor. Cerebral vasospasm. Amsterdam: Elsevier Science Publishers BV; 1993. p. 341–4.

[35] Zubkov AY, Lewis AI, Scalzo D, et al. Morphologic changes after percutaneous transluminal angioplasty. Surg Neurol 1999;51:399–403.

[36] Honma Y, Fujiwara T, Irie K, et al. Morphological changes in human cerebral arteries after percutaneous transluminal angioplasty for vasospasm caused by subarachnoid hemorrhage. Neurosurgery 1995; 36:1073–80.

[37] Yamamoto Y, Smith RR, Bernanke DH. Mechanism of action of balloon angioplasty in cerebral vasospasm. Neurosurgery 1992;30:1–5.

[38] Milburn JM, Moran CJ, Cross DT III, et al. Increase in diameters of vasospastic intracranial arteries by intraarterial papaverine administration. J Neurosurg 1998;88:38–42.

[39] Kaku Y, Yonekawa Y, Tsukahara T, et al. Superselective intra-arterial infusion of papaverine for the treatment of cerebral vasospasm after subarachnoid hemorrhage. J Neurosurg 1992;77:842–7.

[40] Kassell NF, Helm G, Simmons N, et al. Treatment of cerebral vasospasm with intra-arterial papaverine. J Neurosurg 1992;77:848–52.

[41] Marks MP, Steinberg GK, Lane B. Intraarterial papaverine for the treatment of vasospasm. AJNR Am J Neuroradiol 1993;14:822–6.

[42] Clouston JE, Numaguchi Y, Zoarski GH, et al. Intraarterial papaverine infusion for cerebral vasospasm after subarachnoid hemorrhage. AJNR Am J Neuroradiol 1995;16:27–38.

[43] McAuliffe W, Townsend M, Eskridge JM, et al. Intracranial pressure changes induced during papaverine infusion for treatment of vasospasm. J Neurosurg 1995;83:430–4.

[44] Yoshimura S, Tsukahara T, Hashimoto N, et al. Intra-arterial infusion of papaverine combined with intravenous administration of high-dose nicardipine for cerebral vasospasm. Acta Neurochir (Wien) 1995;135:186–90.

[45] Sawada M, Hashimoto N, Tsukahara T, et al. Effectiveness of intra-arterially infused papaverine solutions of various concentrations for the treatment of cerebral vasospasm. Acta Neurochir (Wien) 1997; 139:706–11.

[46] Cross DT III, Moran CJ, Angtuaco EE, et al. Intracranial pressure monitoring during intraarterial papaverine infusion for cerebral vasospasm. AJNR Am J Neuroradiol 1998;19:1319–23.

[47] Polin RS, Hansen CA, German P, et al. Intra-arterially administered papaverine for the treatment of symptomatic cerebral vasospasm. Neurosurgery 1998;42:1256–64.

[48] Fandino J, Kaku Y, Schuknecht B, et al. Improvement of cerebral oxygenation patterns and metabolic validation of superselective intraarterial infusion of papaverine for the treatment of cerebral vasospasm. J Neurosurg 1998;89:93–100.

[49] Firlik KS, Kaufmann AM, Firlik AD, et al. Intra-arterial papaverine for the treatment of cerebral vasospasm following aneurysmal subarachnoid hemorrhage. Surg Neurol 1999;51:66–74.

[50] Zervas NT, Ogilvy CS. Cerebral vasospasm: current clinical management and results. Clin Neurosurg 1999;45:167–76.

[51] Vajkoczy P, Horn P, Bauhuf C, et al. Effect of intra-arterial papaverine on regional cerebral blood flow in hemodynamically relevant cerebral vasospasm. Stroke 2001;32:498–505.

[52] Andaluz N, Tomsick TA, Tew JM Jr, et al. Indications for endovascular therapy for refractory vasospasm after aneurysmal subarachnoid hemorrhage: experience at the University of Cincinnati. Surg Neurol 2002;58:131–8.

[53] Liu JK, Tenner MS, Gottfried ON, et al. Efficacy of multiple intraarterial papaverine infusions for improvement in cerebral circulation time in patients with recurrent cerebral vasospasm. J Neurosurg 2004;100:414–21.

[54] Varsos VG, Liszczak TM, Han DH, et al. Delayed cerebral vasospasm is not reversible by aminophylline, nifedipine, or papaverine in a "two-hemorrhage" canine model. J Neurosurg 1983;58:11–7.

[55] Vorkapic P, Bevan RD, Bevan JA. Longitudinal time course of reversible and irreversible components of chronic cerebrovasospasm of the rabbit basilar artery. J Neurosurg 1991;74:951–5.

[56] Macdonald RL, Zhang J, Sima B, et al. Papaverine-sensitive vasospasm and arterial contractility and compliance after subarachnoid hemorrhage in dogs. Neurosurgery 1995;37:962–7.

[57] Fujiwara N, Honjo Y, Ohkawa M, et al. Intra-arterial infusion of papaverine in experimental cerebral vasospasm. AJNR Am J Neuroradiol 1997;18: 255–62.

[58] Carhuapoma JR, Qureshi AI, Tamargo RJ, et al. In-tra-arterial papaverine-induced seizures: case report and review of the literature. Surg Neurol 2001;56:159–63.

[59] Tsurushima H, Kamezaki T, Nagatomo Y, et al. Complications associated with intraarterial administration of papaverine for vasospasm following subarachnoid hemorrhage—two case reports. Neurol Med Chir (Tokyo) 2000;40:112–5.

[60] Numaguchi Y, Zoarski GH, Clouston JE, et al. Repeat intra-arterial papaverine treatment for recurrent cerebral vasospasm after subarachnoid hemorrhage. Neuroradiology 1997;39:751–9.

[61] Barr JD, Mathis JM, Horton JA. Transient severe brain stem depression during intraarterial papaverine infusion for cerebral vasospasm. AJNR Am J Neuroradiol 1994;15:719–23.

[62] Mathis JM, DeNardo A, Jensen ME, et al. Transient neurologic events associated with intraarterial papaverine infusion for subarachnoid hemorrhage-induced vasospasm. AJNR Am J Neuroradiol 1994;15:1671–4.

[63] Mathis JM, DeNardo AJ, Thibault L, et al. In vitro evaluation of papaverine hydrochloride incompatibilities: a simulation of intraarterial infusion for cerebral vasospasm. AJNR Am J Neuroradiol 1994;15:1665–70.

[64] Mathis JM, Jensen ME, Dion JE. Technical considerations on intra-arterial papaverine hydrochloride for cerebral vasospasm. Neuroradiology 1997;39:90–8.

[65] Smith WS, Dowd CF, Johnston SC, et al. Neurotoxicity of intra-arterial papaverine preserved with chlorobutanol used for the treatment of cerebral vasospasm after aneurysmal subarachnoid hemorrhage. Stroke 2004;35:518–22.

[66] Flamm ES, Adams HP Jr, Beck DW, et al. Dose-escalation study of intravenous nicardipine in patients with aneurysmal subarachnoid hemorrhage. J Neurosurg 1988;68:393–400.

[67] Haley EC Jr, Kassell NF, Torner JC. A randomized controlled trial of high-dose intravenous nicardipine in aneurysmal subarachnoid hemorrhage. A report of the Cooperative Aneurysm Study. J Neurosurg 1993;78:537–47.

[68] Haley EC Jr, Kassell NF, Torner JC. A randomized trial of nicardipine in subarachnoid hemorrhage: angiographic and transcranial Doppler ultrasound results. A report of the Cooperative Aneurysm Study. J Neurosurg 1993;78:548–53.

[69] Haley EC Jr, Kassell NF, Torner JC, et al. A randomized trial of two doses of nicardipine in aneurysmal subarachnoid hemorrhage. A report of the Cooperative Aneurysm Study. J Neurosurg 1994; 80:788–96.

[70] Badjatia N, Topcuoglu MA, Pryor JC, et al. Preliminary experience with intra-arterial nicardipine as a treatment for cerebral vasospasm. AJNR Am J Neuroradiol 2004;25:819–26.

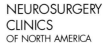

NEUROSURGERY
CLINICS
OF NORTH AMERICA

Neurosurg Clin N Am 16 (2005) 517–540

Antiplatelet Therapy in Neuroendovascular Therapeutics

David Fiorella, MD, PhD[a],*, Lucie Thiabolt, PharmD[b],
Felipe C. Albuquerque, MD[c], Vivek R. Deshmukh, MD[c],
Cameron G. McDougall, MR[c], Peter A. Rasmussen, MD[a]

[a]*Cleveland Clinic Foundation, 9500 Euclid Avenue, S80, Cleveland, OH 44195, USA*
[b]*Boston Scientific Neurovascular, 47900 Bayside Parkway, Freemont, CA 94538, USA*
[c]*Barrow Neurological Institute, 350 West Thomas Road, Phoenix, AZ 85013, USA*

The rapid proliferation of catheter-based devices and neuroendovascular techniques has resulted in an exponential growth in the spectrum of neurologic disease processes that are amenable to percutaneous endovascular therapy. As the scope of pathologic conditions treated by the endovascular neuroradiologist and neurosurgeon broadens, so does the required knowledge base that forms the foundation for rationale decision making and optimal patient management.

Antithrombotic pharmacotherapy currently represents a critical component of this evolving neuroendovascular knowledge base. The importance of optimal antithrombotic therapy should continue to increase in the coming years as carotid stenting emerges as an alternative to endarterectomy, as flexible self-expandable stents for the treatment of intracranial atherosclerotic disease are introduced, and as continued progress is made with respect to the development of intracranial stents to treat cerebral aneurysms.

Agents from all the major classes of antithrombotic drugs, including (1) anticoagulants (heparinoids, warfarin, and related compounds), (2) antiplatelet agents (aspirin, thiopyridines, and IIb/IIIa inhibitors), and (3) fibrinolytics, are used routinely during neuroendovascular procedures. In addition, new agents and new classes of agents with different mechanisms of action (eg, direct thrombin inhibitors like hirudin and bivalirudin) are being continuously added to the armamentarium. Correspondingly, antithrombotic pharmacotherapy represents a perpetually evolving and increasingly complex field.

The myriad of neurologic disease processes that may be addressed endovascularly (eg, aneurysms, arteriovenous malformations [AVMs], and fistulae) are relatively uncommon (in comparison to coronary atheromatous disease), and each category comprises a broad, complex, and heterogeneous collection of lesions. For these reasons, large multicenter trials designed to examine different antithrombotic regimens in neuroendovascular intervention are much more difficult to orchestrate. For this reason, the rationale behind the application of antithrombotic agents in neuroendovascular procedures is based almost exclusively on extrapolations of existing data derived from preventative and interventional cardiology and stroke trials. Although these studies can provide some guidance, fundamental differences with respect to the nature of the disease processes treated and the clinical context in which intervention is undertaken often limit direct translation and application.

In many ways, achieving an optimal level of anticoagulation and platelet inhibition in the context of neuroendovascular intervention is considerably more complex. The brain is an unforgiving end organ, and even relatively minor thromboembolic events may have disastrous clinical implications. The most common disease processes addressed involve acutely hemorrhagic or potentially hemorrhagic vascular lesions that require the

---

* Corresponding author.
  E-mail address: fioreld@ccf.org (D. Fiorella).

operator to negotiate a precarious balance between the prevention of thrombosis and the provocation of hemorrhage. Often, the most demanding decisions regarding antithrombotic therapy must be made emergently on a case by case basis (eg, the management of an acute thromboembolic complication arising in the setting of the embolization of a ruptured aneurysm). For these reasons, a complete understanding of the pharmacology of the existing agents as well as the data available regarding the applications of these agents in different clinical scenarios is required to develop a rational antithrombotic strategy for any given situation.

Platelets represent the predominant component of arterial thrombi and form in response to stimuli like endothelial injury, turbulent blood flow with associated high wall shear stress, or the introduction of an intravascular foreign body. Correspondingly, it follows that platelet inhibition represents the cornerstone of antithrombotic therapy in neuroendovascular intervention.

Mechanisms of platelet aggregation

Adhesion-activation-secretion-aggregation sequence

Platelets are anucleate blood cells with a tremendous capacity for interaction with their surrounding vascular environment. Platelets contain storage granules that hold multiple chemokines, cytokines, and growth factors. In addition, platelets can synthesize bioactive prostaglandins from membrane phospholipids.

In the resting state, the intact endothelium releases inhibitory factors, such as prostacyclin (PGI_2) and nitric oxide (NO), which function to maintain platelets in a nonactivated state (Fig. 1A). After the introduction of a stimulus, a cascade of events begins, which ultimately results in thrombus formation. This cascade consists of platelet adhesion, activation, secretion, and, finally, aggregation (see Fig. 1). The most common and well-understood stimulus is endothelial injury. High wall shear stress or the introduction of an intravascular foreign body represents additional stimuli that can also activate the process of platelet aggregation.

When an endothelial injury exposes thrombogenic collagen and subendothelial matrix, platelets adhere to the injured surface primarily via the interactions between the platelet surface Ib receptor with von Willebrand's factor (vWF) bound to the exposed collagen (see Fig. 1B). These

adherent platelets spread to form a monolayer along the surface of the injured endothelium. The adherent platelets become activated after adhesion. Endothelial injury also exposes tissue factor (TF) to the bloodstream. TF is expressed exclusively by cells (eg, fibroblasts) that are not in contact with the blood under normal circumstances. Exposed TF binds factor VIIa, leading to activation of the intrinsic and extrinsic coagulation pathways that ultimately results in thrombin formation. Thrombin, in addition to converting fibrinogen to fibrin monomers, functions as a potent platelet agonist, resulting in further platelet activation. The activated platelets secrete additional soluble agonists that are prepackaged in storage granules (including ADP, calcium, and serotonin [5-HT]) and synthesize and secrete thromboxane A_2 (TXA_2). These substances all result in the further amplification of platelet activation (see Fig. 1C). Platelet activation by this myriad of agonists results in the stimulation of multiple different intracellular signaling pathways. These pathways all ultimately converge to induce a conformational change in the platelet surface glycoprotein (GP) IIb/IIIa receptor. This conformational change converts the IIb/IIIa receptor from a quiescent low-affinity state to an activated high-affinity binding site for fibrinogen and vWF. The stronger platelet agonists (ie, thrombin, collagen) also recruit additional GP IIb/IIIa receptors from the intracellular storage pool to the platelet surface.

The binding of the active platelet IIb/IIIa receptor to fibrinogen (and vWF) results in the formation of platelet-platelet and platelet-matrix adhesive interactions and the formation of a stable, larger platelet aggregate at the site of injury (see Fig. 1E). Although there is a significant level of redundancy built into the cascade of platelet activation, the binding of the IIb/IIIa receptor to fibrinogen (or vWF) represents the final common pathway to platelet aggregation, and thus the formation of stable thrombus. As this stable platelet aggregate forms, insoluble fibrin monomers begin precipitating around the aggregated platelets and eventually become cross-linked to form a more permanent thrombus.

Interaction of blood with intravascular foreign bodies: catheters, coils, and stents

The response of flowing arterial blood to an intravascular foreign body is incompletely understood. Within seconds after introduction, plasma proteins, predominantly fibrinogen, adhere

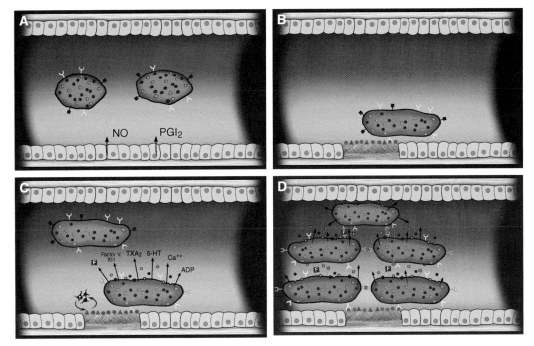

Fig. 1. (*A*) In the resting state, intact endothelial cells release factors like NO and PGI$_2$ to maintain platelets in their inactive state. (*B*) When the endothelium is injured, the breech exposes thrombogenic collagen and subendothelial matrix, which binds vWF (orange circles). (*C*) The platelet surface Ib receptor (yellow receptor) then binds vWF. These adherent platelets spread to form a monolayer along the surface of the injured endothelium. Endothelial injury also exposes TF (green triangles) to the bloodstream. Exposed TF binds factor VIIa, leading to activation of the intrinsic and extrinsic coagulation pathways that ultimately results in thrombin formation. Thrombin, in addition to converting fibrinogen to fibrin monomers, functions as a potent platelet agonist, resulting in further platelet activation. The activated platelets secrete additional soluble agonists that are prepackaged in storage granules (including ADP, calcium, and 5-HT) and synthesize and secrete TXA$_2$. (*D*) These substances all result in the further amplification of platelet activation. Platelet activation by this myriad of agonists results in the stimulation of multiple different intracellular signaling pathways. These pathways all ultimately converge to induce a conformational change in the platelet surface GP IIb/IIIa receptor. This conformational change converts the IIb/IIIa receptor from a quiescent low-affinity state (dark blue receptor) to an activated high-affinity binding site (light blue receptor) for fibrinogen (purple squares) and vWF. The stronger platelet agonists (ie, thrombin, collagen) also recruit additional GP IIb/IIIa receptors from the intracellular storage pool to the platelet surface. The binding of the active platelet IIb/IIIa receptor to fibrinogen (and vWF) results in the formation of platelet-platelet and platelet-matrix adhesive interactions and the formation of stable larger platelet aggregate at the site of injury.

to the surface of the foreign body [1]. These adsorbed proteins, probably in concert with turbulent flow and/or shear stress at the interface between the foreign body and bloodstream, result in platelet adhesion and varying degrees of platelet activation, secretion, and aggregation. Platelet adhesion begins within minutes, forming a layer over the implant during the initial 15 to 90 minutes of contact. Platelet activation may progress, resulting in the formation of platelet aggregates, the activation of blood coagulation, and thrombosis. Alternatively, the implant may undergo a process termed *passivation* and become resistant to further platelet attachment.

The degree of platelet aggregation and thrombosis depends on the characteristics of the implant, including its chemical composition, surface charge, and topography, as well as the local hemodynamic environment, specifically, the associated level of shear stress.

The mechanism of introduction also contributes to this process. During the electrolytic detachment of Guglielmi detachable coils (GDCs), negatively charged blood constituents, particularly platelets and red blood cells, are attracted by the positive charge induced within the platinum coil during detachment. This process of electrothrombosis is theorized to provide a significant contribution to acute occlusion of aneurysms during GDC embolization. Coils detached by other mechanisms would not be expected to induce this effect. A similar disparity is recognized with respect to stenting. The deployment of a balloon-expandable stent for the treatment of atheromatous stenosis is expected to induce significant endothelial injury and subsequent platelet activation. Conversely, the deployment of a low radial force self-expanding intracranial stent (eg, Neuroform; Boston Scientific, Freemont, California) for aneurysm treatment should leave the underlying endothelium relatively intact. Although the introduction of a stent in either scenario could result in in situ thrombosis, this would be expected to occur much more frequently in the context of an endothelial injury induced by a high radial force stent. The consequences of introducing a low radial force self-expanding stent into the cerebral vasculature are largely uncharacterized at this point.

Pharmacology of antiplatelet agents

Aspirin

Mechanism of action

The initial activation of platelets results in the activation of phospholipase A_2, leading to the liberation of arachidonic acid (AA) from membrane phospholipids. AA is immediately converted by cyclo-oxygenase (COX-1) to prostaglandin G_2 (PGG_2) and PGH_2 and then to TXA_2 by thromboxane synthase (TS). TXA_2 is then released from the platelet to participate in a platelet receptor–mediated positive feedback loop, which plays a critical role in the further amplification of regional platelet activation. TXA_2 also functions to recruit additional platelets to the site of thrombus formation and induces local vasoconstriction. Aspirin irreversibly inactivates COX-1 through the acetylation of a serine residue at position 529, thus blocking the conversion of AA to PGG_2 and PGH_2 and, ultimately, the production of TXA_2 (Fig. 2). Platelets lack the synthetic machinery to generate new COX-1. Therefore, this inhibition of TXA_2 synthesis persists for the lifetime of the platelet [2].

Aspirin also has effects on vascular endothelial cells, in which the blockade of COX activity inhibits the synthesis of prostacyclin, a prostaglandin that functions to decrease platelet activation. These effects are typically seen only at higher aspirin doses at which the activity of COX-1 and COX-2 are inhibited. This phenomenon has been termed the *aspirin dilemma* and has led to the hypothesis that an optimal aspirin dose could provide maximal inhibition of TXA_2 synthesis with minimal disruption of the production of PGI_2. In addition, this phenomenon may explain the relatively decreased efficacy of aspirin administered in higher doses [3]. Unlike platelets, vascular endothelial cells have the synthetic machinery to generate new COX enzyme; thus, the inhibition of PGI_2 synthesis is likely to be fully recovered within the interval between the once-daily doses of aspirin administered for platelet inhibition [4].

Pharmacokinetics

The onset of antiplatelet activity after an oral dose of aspirin is remarkably fast. Serum thromboxane B_2 levels (a marker of TXA_2 production) are significantly reduced as early as 5 minutes after oral administration, with the maximum effect occurring within 30 to 60 minutes and remaining stable for 24 hours. The rapid rate of onset has been attributed to the acetylation of COX-1 in platelets within the presystemic portal circulation [4,5].

Dose

Aspirin has a myriad of different effects in addition to its antiplatelet activity, functioning as an analgesic, antipyretic, and anti-inflammatory agent. These effects all exhibit different dose-response relations with the lowest doses required to achieve platelet inhibition. Ex vivo studies of platelet inhibition have demonstrated that similar levels of inhibition can be achieved with daily aspirin doses ranging from 30 to 325 mg [4,5]. In a large meta-analysis, the Antithrombotic Trialists Collaboration found no evidence to support high-dose aspirin therapy. The meta-analysis demonstrated that doses of 75 to 150 mg (32% reduction), 160 to 325 mg (26% reduction), and 500 to 1500 mg (19% reduction) produced similar reductions in vascular events. In this same meta-analysis, doses of less than 75 mg (13% reduction) demonstrated a significantly smaller beneficial effect. In the Aspirin and Carotid Endarterectomy Trial, lower doses of aspirin (81 or 325 mg) resulted in lower rates of stroke, death, and myocardial infarction (MI) than higher (625–1300 mg) dosing regimens at 3 months [3].

Taken together, the available data would suggest that an aspirin dose between 81 and 325 mg would provide an optimal risk profile. If the lower range is to be used (ie, 81 mg/d), the operator should consider the administration of a 162- to

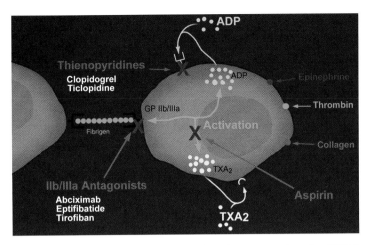

Fig. 2. Mechanisms of action of antiplatelet agents. Aspirin functions to acetylate the COX-1 enzyme irreversibly, thereby blocking the synthesis of TXA_2. Clopidogrel functions to irreversibly block the P2Y12 receptor (light blue). ADP and TXA_2 represent only two of multiple soluble agonists that function to activate platelets. Although the soluble agonist pathways that lead to platelet activation are highly redundant, IIb/IIIa receptor activation represents the final common pathway on which all these pathways converge to enable platelet aggregation and the formation of a stable platelet thrombus. The IIb/IIIa receptor antagonists function irreversibly (abciximab) or reversibly (eptifibatide, tirofiban) to block this component of the platelet aggregation cascade. (Adapted from Steinhubl SR. Aspirin and thienopyridines, transcatheter cardiovascular therapeutics, expert presentations pool. 2004; with permission.)

325-mg loading dose so that a therapeutic level of antiplatelet activity can be achieved immediately.

Resistance

Aspirin resistance is a significant problem that has been recognized recently as tests for the adequacy of platelet blockade have become more available. Between 5% and 40% of patients are resistant to the antiplatelet effects of standard doses of aspirin [6,7]. The incidence of aspirin resistance has been found to be related to aspirin dose. In a study of patients with previous ischemic stroke on aspirin therapy, platelet function testing with a platelet function analyzer (PFA)-100 system demonstrated 56% resistance at an 81 mg daily dose and 28% resistance at a 325 mg dose [8]. These same authors reported that 65% of patients taking enteric coated aspirin had normal platelet function test results. In addition, aspirin resistance may progressively develop over time with long-term therapy. Pulcinelli et al [9] observed a significant reduction in platelet sensitivity to aspirin therapy over a 24-month period.

A growing volume of data suggests that aspirin resistance has significant clinical implications. Gum et al [6] reported a three times higher risk of death, MI, and cerebrovascular accident (CVA) in stable cardiovascular patients over an approximately 2-year period. Chen et al [7] found aspirin-resistant patients to have a three times greater risk of having creatine kinase (CK)-MB elevations after nonemergent percutaneous coronary intervention (PCI). In patients with a prior stroke, those with aspirin resistance were 89% more likely to have a recurrent cerebrovascular accident within 2 years [10]. After peripheral intervention, an increase in arterial reocclusion has been observed in a cohort of aspirin nonresponders [11].

Although no studies currently exist, similar implications should be anticipated for neuroendovascular patients undergoing procedures requiring stent deployment or angioplasty. A priori knowledge of aspirin resistance could significantly influence the treatment plan, particularly in those cases in which other reasonable therapeutic options exist (eg, carotid endarterectomy versus carotid stenting, balloon-assisted versus stent-assisted aneurysm embolization).

Thienopyridines: clopidogrel and ticlopidine

Mechanism of action

Clopidogrel (Plavix) and ticlopidine (Ticlid) are the two available thienopyridines that have been routinely applied for use as antiplatelet agents. Both agents have no activity in vitro because they require hepatic transformation to active metabolites that mediate the antiplatelet effect. The active metabolites irreversibly inhibit ADP from binding to its platelet surface P2Y12 receptor (see Fig. 2). This blockade prevents the soluble platelet agonist ADP from stimulating activation of the intracellular second-messenger (adenylate cyclase) system, which functions to amplify regional platelet activation by stimulating secretion and ultimately modulates the conversion of the GP IIb/IIIa receptor to its high-affinity state.

Ticlopidine use has declined substantially over the past decade because of the associated side effect of bone marrow depression, with neutropenia occurring in 2.4% of patients, and the emergence of clopidogrel as an adequate substitute [12]. In the Clopidogrel Aspirin Stent International Cooperative Study (CLASSICS), a direct comparison of ticlopidine and clopidogrel administered in combination with aspirin, clopidogrel demonstrated a superior safety profile and comparable efficacy in preventing thrombotic complications after coronary stenting [13]. Studies of the pharmacokinetics of both agents indicate that clopidogrel also demonstrates a more prompt onset of maximal platelet inhibition in comparison to ticlopidine [14]. Currently, the use of ticlopidine is largely restricted to patients who are intolerant of clopidogrel. For this reason, the remainder of this section focuses on the pharmacology of clopidogrel.

Pharmacokinetics and dosing: clopidogrel

Clopidogrel is rapidly absorbed and quickly metabolized, with extremely low plasma concentrations of the drug measured in patients on daily therapy [15]. The active metabolite(s) produce an irreversible alteration of the ADP binding site, and, subsequently, the effect persists for the duration of the platelet's lifespan, with 7 days required for the return of normal platelet function after therapeutic levels are attained.

The time required to establish maximally therapeutic levels of platelet inhibition with clopidogrel is dependent on the dosing regimen used [16]. If a standard daily dose of 75 mg is administered without a loading dose, significant levels of platelet inhibition can be measured at 12 to 24 hours. Daily doses of 75 mg produce only 25% to 30% inhibition at 48 hours, however. An average of 5 days (range: 3–7 days) is required to achieve maximal steady-state levels (50%–60%) of platelet inhibition at this dose [17,18]. If a loading dose (300–600 mg) is administered, however, maximal levels of inhibition are achieved

within 2 to 6 hours and remain relatively stable for up to 48 hours [17,19,20]. In the CREDO study, patients who received the 300-mg clopidogrel loading dose 6 hours or more before the procedure had a 38.6% reduction in death, MI, or urgent target vessel revascularization at 1 month, whereas no benefit was observed in patients receiving the loading dose before the 6-hour time point [21].

Resistance

The efficacy of clopidogrel differs between patients with a significant incidence of resistance. Unlike aspirin, clopidogrel resistance has been classified as a binary as well as a graded phenomenon by different investigators. Resistance is measured by determining the degree of reduction in ADP-induced platelet aggregation. Gurbel et al [22] observed resistance in 31% of patients at 24 hours and 5 days, decreasing to 15% at 30 days after a 300 mg loading dose of clopidogrel and a dose of 75 mg/d after that. When divided into subcategories, Muller et al [23] reported that 5% to 11% were nonresponders and 9% to 26% were semiresponders, depending on the dose of ADP used to stimulate platelet aggregation. Lau et al [24] reported rates of clopidogrel resistance in 22% of patients and 16% of volunteers, with an additional 23% of patients and 12% of volunteers categorized as "low" responders.

Similar to aspirin, clopidogrel resistance has been demonstrated to have significant clinical implications. For example, individual variability in response to clopidogrel in the setting of PCI after MI was found to predict an increased risk of recurrent cardiovascular events [25].

Unlike aspirin, clopidogrel resistance does not seem to develop with time. Thus, if a patient is confirmed to be responsive initially, a durable antiplatelet effect can be anticipated with long-term administration [26]. This durability may account for the added benefit observed when clopidogrel is added to supplement long-term aspirin therapy.

The mechanisms of clopidogrel resistance are incompletely understood. The leading hypothesis is that individual differences in hepatic metabolism result in variable rates of conversion of the clopidogrel to its active metabolite [24].

Reversal

As with aspirin, platelet inhibition by the thienopyridines is durable for the lifetime of the platelet. Platelet function gradually returns to normal, via platelet turnover, over a period of 7 days after the last dose of clopidogrel is administered. Correspondingly, immediate reversal can only be achieved with a platelet transfusion.

Dipyridamole

Mechanism of action

The mechanism by which dipyridamole inhibits platelet activity is poorly understood. Hypotheses include increases in intracellular cyclic AMP levels via the inhibition of phosphodiesterase or the blockade of adenosine uptake, direct stimulation of PGI_2 synthesis or inhibition of PGI_2 degradation, and the potentiation of the effects of NO. The concentrations of the agent required to achieve these effects are far greater than those achieved at conventional dosing regimens, however [27].

Pharmacokinetics and dosing

The pharmacokinetics of dipyridamole are also complex. The conventional formulations of the agent result in poor systemic bioavailability. As such, an extended-release formulation (200 mg) has been introduced and is available in combination with low-dose aspirin (25 mg). The half-life of the dipyridamole is 10 hours, which forms the basis for a twice-daily dosing regimen in the existing clinical studies [28]. Because of its vasodilatory effects and potential to provoke a coronary steal phenomenon when used as a pharmacologic stress agent, there has been some concern about the routine use of dipyridamole in patients with coronary artery disease (CAD) [29].

Resistance

We are aware of no studies that have evaluated patients for dipyridamole resistance.

IIb/IIIa inhibitors

Mechanism of action

The IIb/IIIA inhibitors block platelet aggregation by preventing fibrinogen and other adhesion molecules (vWF) from binding to the IIb/IIIa integrin on platelets. There are two general classes of antagonists: the irreversible antagonist abciximab (Reopro) and the reversible antagonists eptifibatide and tirofiban. Abciximab is a monoclonal antibody that binds irreversibly to the IIb/IIIa receptor at the β-chain of the integrin. Eptifibatide (Integrilin) and tirofiban (Aggrastat) are peptides that mimic the naturally occurring arginine-glycine-aspartic acid (RGD) sequence that is avidly bound by the IIb/IIIa receptor. This RGD binding site mediates the binding of vWF, vitronectin, fibronectin, and fibrinogen to platelets. Eptifibatide and tirofiban compete with these factors for binding at the RGD site, functioning as reversible competitive inhibitors of the IIb/IIIa receptor. By eliminating the function of the IIb/IIIa receptor, these agents block the final common pathway of platelet function—platelet aggregation. At approximately 80% IIb/IIIa receptor blockade, platelet aggregation is nearly completely abolished, and at levels greater than 90%, platelet function is ablated to the point that bleeding times become markedly elevated [30].

In addition to its effects at the platelet IIb/IIIa receptor, abciximab binds to the vitronectin receptor (vascular smooth muscle and endothelial cells) and the integrin Mac-1 (activated neutrophils and monocytes). The consequences of these additional receptor interactions remain to be elucidated; however, some have hypothesized that these interactions may play a role in decreasing the inflammatory reaction that follows angioplasty or stenting, thus limiting subsequent intimal hyperplasia.

Side effects

All three IIb/IIIa inhibitors have the potential to induce thrombocytopenia. This occurs at a slightly higher rate with abciximab (up to 6.5%) in comparison to the competitive antagonists [31]. Thrombocytopenia induced by IIb/IIIa inhibitors is usually quickly reversed by stopping the drug. Typically, complete recovery evolves over several days.

Pharmacokinetics and dose: abciximab

Abciximab, a monoclonal antibody, is a large molecule with extremely high affinity for platelet IIb/IIIa receptors. Correspondingly, the plasma half-life of the free drug is short, approximately 10 minutes, because the agent binds immediately to circulating platelets. The agent not bound to platelet receptors is quickly cleared from the circulation. Once bound to platelets, the dissociation time is long and the molecule remains biologically active on the surface of platelets for 12 to 14 hours. These characteristics result in a rapid onset of action and a slow reversal of activity after cessation of administration. After the administration of a bolus and infusion of abciximab, 28% occupation of the IIb/IIIa receptors is sustained at 8 days, declining to 13% at 15 days.

Abciximab is typically administered as a loading dose of 0.25 mg/kg, followed by an infusion at 0.125 μg/kg/min (maximum of 10 μg/min) for 12 hours. If the bolus is given alone, bleeding times recover to near-normal values by 12 hours, with platelet aggregation returning to greater than 50% of baseline within 24 to 48 hours in almost all patients. If the infusion is administered, platelet inactivation is maintained throughout the duration of the infusion.

Pharmacokinetics and dose: eptifibatide and tirofiban

Eptifibatide, a synthetic peptide, is a structural analogue of barbourin, a snake venom disintegrin polypeptide. Tirofiban is a nonpeptide tyrosin derivative also based on the structure of a known disintegrin polypeptide. These agents have less affinity than abciximab for the IIb/IIIa receptor, and their binding to the receptor is reversible. Eptifibatide, in particular, is a low-affinity agonist for the IIb/IIIa receptor. Both compounds demonstrate a rapid dissociation from the receptor (seconds). Correspondingly, after cessation of administration, platelet function returns rapidly to normal. Both agents are cleared through the kidneys, and as such, the effects of these agents may persist longer in patients with renal failure. The plasma half-time of both agents is approximately 1.5 hours in patients with normal renal function. Bleeding times begin to return toward normal shortly (within 15 minutes) after the discontinuation of eptifibatide, with a return to greater than half of the normal platelet aggregation response within 4 hours. Bleeding times also return to normal within approximately 4 hours after discontinuation of the tirofiban infusion, with platelet aggregation inhibition declining to levels less than 50% at this time point.

The Platelet Aggregation and Receptor Occupancy with Integrilin (PRIDE) study demonstrated that a 180 μg/kg bolus of eptifibatide followed by a 2.0 μg/kg/min infusion for 12 hours consistently resulted in greater than 90% platelet inhibition within 5 minutes. This effect was decreased at 1 hour, however, and did not return to the targeted therapeutic level until a steady state was reached at 8 to 24 hours. For this reason, it is currently recommended that two boluses (180 μg/kg) be administered 10 minutes apart, followed by a continuous 2.0 μg/kg/min infusion to achieve a more stable therapeutic effect [32,33]. Tirofiban is administered as a 10-μg/kg bolus, followed by an infusion of 0.15 μg/kg/min for 12 hours. This

regimen results in a mean inhibition of platelet aggregation (ADP, 5 μmol/L) of 96% at 5 minutes, 100% at 2 hours, and 95% at the end of the infusion [34].

When IIb/IIIa receptor inhibitors are used in conjunction with heparin, the dose of heparin should be decreased (50–70 U/kg) slightly, because existing literature indicates an increased risk of bleeding without significantly increased efficacy [35,36].

Resistance

The therapeutic window for these agents is narrow, because the occupation of approximately 80% of IIb/IIIa receptors is required for clinically effective inhibition of platelet aggregation; however, greater than 90% inhibition may result in excessive bleeding complications [37]. The number of platelet receptors available for binding varies with the relative state of platelet activation [38]. In addition, the actual platelet counts and, subsequently, the number of receptors vary quite substantially across patients [39]. As such, determining a universal dose of IIb/IIIa inhibitors for any given patient is challenging.

In a study directly comparing the efficacy of all three agents in the setting of high-risk PCI, it was determined that only 52% of patients achieved targeted levels of platelet inhibition after administration of the recommended bolus dose of IIb/IIIa inhibitor (41%, 66%, and 49% with tirofiban, eptifibatide, and abciximab, respectively). The remaining 48% of patients required a second half-bolus to achieve the target levels [40]. In the GOLD [41] study, 25% of all patients administered the recommended bolus doses of IIb/IIIa inhibitors did not achieve adequate platelet inhibition and experienced a significantly higher incidence of adverse cardiac events.

Thus, as with aspirin and the thienopyridines, there is substantial variability in the level of platelet function inhibition achieved with standard regimens of GP IIb/IIIa antagonist therapy, and the level of platelet function inhibition is an independent predictor for the risk of complications during PCI.

Reversal of activity

Abciximab has a protracted duration of action, and reversal requires platelet transfusion. The antiplatelet effects of the competitive antagonists abate over a relatively short period if the infusion is discontinued. Although platelet transfusions hasten the return of normal function, they are less effective in this setting, because the competitive antagonists have a short dissociation time and maintain higher plasma concentrations. Fibrinogen supplementation in the form of cryoprecipitate or fresh-frozen plasma represents a useful means by which to achieve reversal of these agents. The increasing concentration of fibrinogen tips the balance of competition at the IIb/IIIa receptor in favor of fibrinogen, counteracting the effects of the circulating IIb/IIIa inhibitors [42].

Comparative clinical efficacy

In a direct comparison, abciximab was superior to tirofiban for the prevention of ischemic events after percutaneous transluminal coronary angioplasty (PTCA) [43]. In a comparison of all three agents in high-risk patients undergoing PTCA, however, no difference in major cardiac events was detected at 30 days [40].

Measurement of antiplatelet activity

In neuroendovascular therapeutics, the ability to assess the status of platelet function rapidly and accurately is critical. Not infrequently, antiplatelet agents must be reversed immediately and completely to accommodate a required surgical intervention (eg, ventriculostomy catheter placement or craniotomy) or in response to a procedural hemorrhagic complication. Alternatively, given the frequency, and associated clinical implications, of antiplatelet agent resistance, adequate platelet inhibition is prerequisite to the safe execution of endovascular procedures requiring the deployment of a device within the parent vessel or when performing angioplasty.

Although several assays are currently available, they have not yet emerged as a routine component in the practice of peripheral, coronary, or endovascular therapeutics at most institutions. In addition, the existing assays have significant limitations. As such, the means by which to achieve accurate and accessible measurements of platelet function continue to evolve.

Bleeding time

The measurement of bleeding time is a universally available and relatively simple technique by which to measure platelet function at the bedside. Although the means of assay differ, all methods require a skin incision, usually made on the earlobe or forearm, of a depth that results in the disruption of capillary loops and small vessels. The normal ranges for bleeding time vary significantly with the type of assay used. The measurement of bleeding time has been criticized as an insensitive, inaccurate, nonspecific, and poorly reproducible measure of platelet function. The irreproducibility of the test result also arises because the measurements are dependent on multiple variables in addition to platelet function, including platelet count, red blood cell count and function, and vessel wall integrity [44].

Optical aggregometry

The current "gold standard" assay for platelet function is agonist-induced aggregation measured by optical aggregometry (turbidometric) in citrated blood samples. This assay measures the increased transmission of light through platelet samples that occurs as platelets aggregate in response to the addition of various soluble agonists and precipitate from the suspension. Different agonists are available to assess the activity of different antiplatelet agents. "Resistance" to a given agent is defined as failure of the agent to inhibit agonist-induced platelet aggregation sufficiently, which is expressed as a percentage of mean aggregation. It is important to note that these are specialized laboratory tests requiring unique expertise; as such, they are not universally available.

Aspirin therapy is typically monitored with the agonists ADP (5–20 μmol/L), AA, or collagen. Aspirin resistance is defined at our institution as a mean aggregation of greater than 70% with ADP (10 μmol/L) and greater than 20% with AA (0.5 mg/mL) [6]. Clopidogrel resistance is typically measured by assessing the platelet response to the agonist ADP (20 μmol/L). Clopidogrel nonresponders, low responders, and responders were defined by a mean aggregation of greater than 90%, 90% to 71%, and less than 70% compared with a preclopidogrel administration baseline, respectively, by Lau et al [24]. IIb/IIIa antagonist resistance is measured by the response of platelets to ADP (5–20 μmol/L) and other agonists (eg, thrombin receptor agonist peptides [TRAPs]). Different studies have used variable criteria to define resistance attributable to methodologic differences in the assays (anticoagulants used in the collected samples and doses of ADP used for the stimulation of platelet aggregation), however [45]. Having said this, initial dose-finding studies used a targeted level of platelet inhibition to 20%

of baseline ADP (20 μmol/L)-induced platelet aggregation [46].

Point-of-care rapid platelet function assay

The Verify Now (Ultegra Rapid Platelet Function Assay) system (Accumetrics, San Diego, California) provides a means by which to measure aspirin, clopidogrel, and IIb/IIIa inhibitor function rapidly, using a citrated whole blood sample, at the bedside (point-of-care monitoring). A Vacutainer containing citrate-anticoagulated blood is inserted in a fully self-contained assay device that contains fibrinogen-coated beads and platelet agonists. If platelet function is impaired in response to a given antiplatelet agent, the fibrinogen-coated beads do not agglutinate and light transmission through the sample does not increase. Different assay devices containing different agonists are available for the assessment of each of the different antiplatelet agents.

For the aspirin test, AA is used as the agonist and the results are reported as aspirin reaction units (ARUs). Aspirin induces a dose-related decrease in ARU using this method. An ARU greater than 550 indicates aspirin nonresponsiveness (the absence of aspirin-induced platelet dysfunction). Correlation with light transmission aggregometry with AA indicated a sensitivity of 100% and a specificity of 91.4% for the determination of aspirin resistance. Assessments of patient reproducibility indicated coefficients of variation of 2.5% (within the same patient) and 12.5% to 15% (between patients), respectively [47]. If the patient is being given a GP IIb/IIIa inhibitor or clopidogrel, the results of the aspirin test reflect not only the effects of aspirin but those of these agents. A patient resistant to aspirin but well treated with clopidogrel and aspirin may have an ARU measurement of less than 550.

The VerifyNow P2Y12 assay is currently available for research use only. This system uses ADP as the platelet agonist in combination with an additional antagonist to confer specificity for the measurement of ADP-induced platelet aggregation occurring through the P2Y12 receptor (the receptor that is blocked by clopidogrel). As such, the result of this assay specifically reflects the efficacy of clopidogrel.

The VerifyNow IIb/IIIa assay device uses TRAP as the platelet agonist. TRAP is the most potent agonist of platelet aggregation and is not affected by aspirin and minimally affected by clopidogrel. The assay reports results in platelet activating units (PAUs), with normal predrug levels ranging between 125 and 330 and therapeutic postdrug levels of less than 44. Results may also be reported as percent inhibition based on the differences between the baseline and postdrug results, with a target level of greater than 90% inhibition used in some studies for PCI [40].

Relevant data from clinical antiplatelet trials

Anti-Thrombotic Trialists Collaboration

The most comprehensive summary of available data regarding the clinical efficacy of antiplatelet therapy comes from the Anti-Thrombotic Trialists Collaboration [48]. This study incorporated data from 287 studies (comprehensive through September 1997) involving 135,000 "high-risk" patients in comparisons of antiplatelet therapy versus controls. High-risk patients were those with acute or previous vascular disease or with significant risk factors for vascular disease. In these patients, allocation to antiplatelet therapy resulted in an overall 22% reduction in the odds ratio of serious vascular events in comparison to controls (17.8% versus 21.4%; $P < 0.001$). They observed a 17% reduction in all vascular mortality, a 33% decrease in nonfatal MI, and a 25% decrease in the rate of stroke. Clopidogrel and ticlopidine were more effective than aspirin, decreasing events by 10% and 12% in comparison to aspirin therapy, respectively. The addition of dipyridamole to aspirin was not found to be beneficial in comparison to aspirin therapy alone. In patients with a history of stroke or transient ischemic attack (TIA), antiplatelet therapy resulted in 36 fewer significant vascular events per 1000, primarily accounted for by a decreased rate of nonfatal stroke (25 of 1000 patients). In these patients, vascular and all-cause mortality were significantly reduced. In patients with acute stroke, antiplatelet therapy reduced vascular events by 11%. This included a reduction in ischemic stroke of 6.9 per 1000 patients, the benefit of which is slightly attenuated by an increased risk of hemorrhagic stroke of 1.9 per 1000 patients.

Clopidogrel Versus Aspirin in Individuals at Risk of Ischemic Events study

With the emergence of clopidogrel as an adequate substitute for ticlopidine, interest arose in determining the relative efficacy of clopidogrel in comparison to aspirin. The Clopidogrel Versus Aspirin in Individuals at Risk of Ischemic Events (CAPRIE) study was a large prospective, randomized, blind, level I comparison of clopidogrel (75 mg, n = 9577) versus aspirin (325, n = 9566) in patients with thrombotic disease (stroke, MI, 35 days old, and symptomatic atherosclerotic peripheral artery disease [PAD]) who were followed for 1 to 3 years for the end points of stroke, MI, and vascular death. These observers reported an 8.7% relative risk reduction (RRR) in favor of clopidogrel, with the number of patients needed to be treated (NNT) over 1 year of 196. The overall benefit can be attributed to the disproportionate benefit observed in patients with PAD (RRR = 23.8, range: 8.9–36.2). No significant differences were observed for patients in the stroke group (RRR = 7.3, range: −5.7–18.7) or MI group (RRR = −3.7, range: −22.1–12.0). More significant benefits were observed in some particularly high-risk subgroups, such as patients with previous coronary artery bypass grafting (RRR = 28.9%, NNT = 16), multiple ischemic events (NNT = 50), multiple vascular beds involved (NNT = 41), diabetes mellitus (NNT = 48 [26.3 if on insulin]), and increased cholesterol (NNT = 77). In addition to the significant reductions in primary end points, there were significant reductions in hospitalization for ischemic events and bleeding events (including gastrointestinal bleeding) for patients on Clopidogrel [49].

Clopidogrel in Unstable Angina to Prevent Recurrent Events and Clopidogrel for the Reduction of Events during Observation studies

The antiplatelet effects of clopidogrel and aspirin are mediated by two different receptors. Correspondingly, it is expected that the two agents together could potentially have a synergistic effect. This was first demonstrated in ex vivo experiments [50] and later evaluated clinically in two large cardiology studies: Clopidogrel in Unstable Angina to Prevent Recurrent Events (CURE) and Clopidogrel for the Reduction of Events during Observation (CREDO).

In the CURE study, patients with acute coronary syndrome were treated with aspirin (75–325 mg/d) and placebo (n = 6303) or clopidogrel (75 mg/d, n = 6259) for 3 to 12 months (average of 9 months). Patients treated with both agents demonstrated lower risks of the combined end points of cardiovascular death, MI, and stroke (9.3% versus

11.4%; $P < 0.0001$; RRR = 20%, NNT = 48) with an increased risk of major bleeding (3.7% versus 2.7%). The beneficial effect of clopidogrel was observed across all doses of aspirin. Bleeding risks increased with increasing doses of aspirin despite the lack of any benefit of increased doses on the combined end points measured [51].

When the subset of CURE patients undergoing PCI were selectively evaluated, the beneficial effects of dual-agent therapy were even more evident, with a 31% reduction ($P = 0.002$) in stroke, death, and MI. This beneficial effect was evident before PCI, 1 month after PCI, and at the end of follow-up (average of 8 months) [52].

In the CREDO study, a randomized placebo-controlled trial, patients who were designated to be at a high likelihood of needing PCI were treated with placebo or a 300 mg clopidogrel loading dose before the anticipated interventional procedure. After the procedure, all patients were maintained on clopidogrel at a dose of 75 mg/d. Patients who received the loading dose of clopidogrel before the procedure were maintained on clopidogrel for 1 year. Patients who received the 300 mg clopidogrel loading dose 6 hours or more before the procedure had a 38.6% reduction in death, MI, or urgent target vessel revascularization at 1 month. No benefit was observed in patients receiving the loading dose before the 6-hour time point. In the group treated with clopidogrel for 1 year, a 27% reduction in the combined end points was observed in comparison to those who were treated for only 1 month.

The PCI CURE and CREDO investigators concluded that the continuation of clopidogrel therapy (in addition to aspirin) for up to 1 year resulted in a significant improvement in patient outcomes [21]. In both studies, however, those patients randomized to long-term clopidogrel therapy were the same as those initially randomized to receive a clopidogrel loading dose before PCI. Correspondingly, it is impossible to determine for certain whether the long-term benefits of dual-agent therapy are attributable to the prevention of complications incurred during the initial intervention or to the prevention of new events by sustained dual-agent antiplatelet inhibition, or both [53]. Currently, this remains a somewhat contentious point in cardiology, although most have gravitated to long-term dual-antiplatelet therapy. This is particularly true in patients receiving drug-eluting coronary stents (DES), because a DES requires a longer period to complete endothelialization. In neuroendovascular therapeutics, the issues surrounding the optimal duration of dual-antiplatelet therapy are further complicated by the results of the MATCH trial.

Aspirin and clopidogrel compared with clopidogrel alone after recent ischemic stroke or transient ischemic attack in high-risk patients

In the prospective, randomized, placebo-controlled, double-blind MATCH trial, patients (n = 7599) at high risk for cerebral ischemia (recent ischemic stroke or TIA and at least one additional vascular risk factor) were treated with clopidogrel (75 mg/d) and aspirin (75 mg/d) or placebo for up to 18 months. A nonsignificant decrease in the primary end points (15.7% and 16.7% for the aspirin and placebo groups, respectively [RRR = −4.6% and −16.3%; *P* = 0.244]) of stroke, MI, vascular death, or rehospitalization for acute ischemia (central nervous system, coronary, or peripheral) was observed with the addition of aspirin to clopidogrel. A 1.3% increase in the rate of life-threatening bleeding was observed in the aspirin group. Thus, although aspirin was ineffective in preventing ischemic events, the addition of aspirin to clopidogrel therapy did result in increased bleeding [54].

Although useful, the results of this trial must be viewed in the context of the population studied. Because of the requirement of a secondary vascular risk factor, 70% of the patients included were diabetic and 54% of patients presented with a lacunar infarct as the qualifying ischemic event. In addition, the subset of patients with CAD were largely excluded from the study given that their cardiologists were hesitant to include patients in a trial that might result in randomization to single-agent antiplatelet therapy. Thus, although the results indicate no significant advantage of adding aspirin to clopidogrel, one must first consider that the results suggested a trend toward a benefit from adding aspirin and then consider that the study population was not composed of the typical patients seen by the neuroendovascular interventionist, who is more frequently consulted for the evaluation of angiographically evident large-vessel disease rather than small-vessel ischemic disease.

A clinical trial of abciximab in elective percutaneous coronary intervention after pretreatment with clopidogrel

In a prospective (2159 patients) randomized trial of abciximab versus placebo in low-risk patients undergoing elective PCI (pretreated with clopidogrel and aspirin), no significant differences in outcomes were observed at 30 days [55]. This trial contradicts the results of multiple other trials that observed a benefit of adding IIb/IIIa inhibitors in patients undergoing PCI.

The initial studies establishing the beneficial effects of IIb/IIIa inhibitors were conducted in high-risk patients. The EPIC study [56] demonstrated a significant reduction (30% RRR) in all adverse ischemic events when an abciximab bolus and infusion were added to conventional heparin and aspirin therapy in high-risk patients (acute MI, recent MI, unstable angina, or high-risk lesions) undergoing PCI. Similarly, the CAPTURE [57] trial demonstrated the efficacy (47% RRR) of abciximab before treatment in patients with unstable angina refractory to conventional therapy undergoing PCI.

These results were then evaluated in a broader group of patients. In the EPISTENT trial [58], an abciximab bolus and infusion significantly (52.9% RRR) reduced adverse ischemic events (death, MI, or urgent revascularization) at 30 days in a less selected group of patients (pretreated with aspirin, ticlopidine, and heparin) undergoing elective or urgent PTCA or stenting. These early benefits were also manifest at 1 year of follow-up as a significant reduction in mortality in patients undergoing stenting with an abciximab bolus and infusion [59]. The IMPACT II [60] and Randomized Efficacy Study of Tirofiban for Outcomes and Restenosis (RESTORE) [61] trials demonstrated similar trends toward improved outcomes after PCI performed with eptifibatide and tirofiban; however, neither study reached significance with respect to a reduction in adverse ischemic events at 30 days. In the European-Australian Stroke Prevention in Reversible Ischemia Trial (ESPRIT) [33], a new dosing regimen of eptifibatide using two boluses followed by an infusion markedly reduced adverse ischemic events at 48 hours in unselected patients (pretreated with aspirin, heparin, and a thienopyridine) undergoing PCI.

Thus, before the Kastrati et al [55] study, the question was not whether to use a IIb/IIIa receptor antagonist as an adjunct to PCI but which one to use. The lack of an additive benefit of abciximab observed by Kastrati et al [55] is most likely attributable to the high clopidogrel loading dose (600 mg) used in this series. It is likely that this aggressive loading dose resulted in a high proportion of patients with therapeutic levels of clopidogrel-induced platelet inhibition at the time of PCI. Correspondingly, these results suggest that if adequate pretreatment with dual-antiplatelet agents is established, the addition of a IIb/IIIa antagonist is likely not beneficial and may expose the patient to an unnecessary risk of a hemorrhagic complication.

Applications of antiplatelet agents in interventional neuroradiology

There are no widely accepted antiplatelet regimens for application in common neuroendovascular scenarios. The agents selected and doses reported vary widely. Frequently, these decisions are based on individual operator experience and practice patterns rather than on an extrapolation of the existing data.

Stent placement

Neuroendovascular stent placement differs from coronary stenting in several important ways. First, a significant percentage of stents are placed not to restore patency to a narrowed artery but to support aneurysm embolization. In these cases, self-expanding stents with low radial force are used, resulting in little, if any, endothelial injury. In all likelihood, much of what is currently understood about the biology of balloon-expandable coronary stents is not applicable in this setting. Second, when stenting is undertaken to augment or re-establish blood flow, the neurovascular end organ (unlike the heart) is susceptible to reperfusion hemorrhage or hemorrhage as a sequela of ischemic injury that occurred before or during the procedure. These differences must be taken into account when designing antiplatelet regimens for these two subsets of patients.

Despite the differences between stenting for atheromatous disease and stenting for aneurysm therapy, the pretreatment and intraprocedural antiplatelet strategies are similar. Both are geared toward preventing acute stent thrombosis and distal thromboembolic complications related to stent deployment. When performed on an elective basis, the existing literature supports pretreatment with aspirin (162–325-mg loading dose at least 2 hours before the procedure, with continued administration of 81 mg/d up to and including the morning of the procedure) and clopidogrel (300–600 mg bolus administered greater than 6 hours before the procedure, with continued administration of 75 mg/d up to and including the morning of the procedure). Although not routinely available at many institutions, optimal practice would include verification of adequate platelet inhibition before initiation of the procedure.

Some investigators have explored the utility of IIb/IIIa inhibitors as adjunctive agents to lower the risk of the thromboembolic complications associated with carotid stenting. In two small patient series reporting experiences using abciximab in the setting of carotid stenting, a significant risk of intracerebral hemorrhage was observed [62,63]. In a later series of studies, these same investigators found eptifibatide to be a safe adjunct to carotid stenting [64,65]. Whether safe or not, the recent data of Kastrati et al [55] regarding the utility of IIb/IIIa inhibitors in coronary stenting would suggest that the application of such agents is not necessary if adequate platelet inhibition is established with aspirin and clopidogrel before treatment. In all likelihood, the routine addition of a IIb/IIIa inhibitor to an effective regimen of dual-antiplatelet therapy poses minimal benefit and may carry with it a significant risk.

For these reasons, we do not routinely use IIb/IIIa inhibitors in conjunction with aspirin and clopidogrel during elective stenting procedures. We reserve the use of these agents for patients with angiographically evident intraprocedural thromboembolic events and for those patients stented without aspirin and clopidogrel pretreatment (Fig. 3). This is often performed emergently in the context of a bailout and/or salvage maneuver or to restore flow to a threatened vascular distribution on an emergent basis (Fig. 4). In these cases, we have administered a 0.25 mg/kg loading bolus of abciximab to establish immediate platelet inhibition. In some cases, we have administered 50% to 100% of the initial bolus intra-arterially, with the remainder of the bolus dose given intravenously. The intra-arterial administration of a portion of the abciximab bolus is intended to achieve a high local concentration of the agent rapidly in the immediate vicinity of the recently deployed stent. If the treatment was undertaken in the setting of an underlying acutely hemorrhagic lesion (eg, a ruptured aneurysm), the patient is administered a loading dose of aspirin (162–325 mg) and clopidogrel (300–600 mg) immediately after the procedure in lieu of a 12-hour abciximab infusion. If the underlying lesion is not acutely hemorrhagic, the abciximab infusion is administered, with the loading doses of aspirin and clopidogrel given immediately after the procedure. Abciximab therapy is best monitored using point-of-care testing to verify adequate levels of platelet inhibition. In this setting, this monitoring

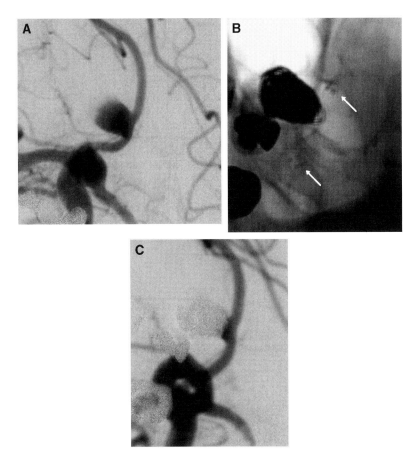

Fig. 3. (*A*) A 76-year-old woman with an unruptured anterior communicating artery complex aneurysm presented for coil embolization. The patient was not pretreated with antiplatelet agents. (*B*) Because of the width of the aneurysm neck, a 2.5-mm × 15-mm Neuroform stent was placed to support coil embolization (white arrows indicate the radiopaque markers delineating the ends of the stent). Immediately preceding deployment of the stent, the patient was administered an intravenous bolus of abciximab (0.25 mg/kg). After the intravenous bolus, the stent was successfully deployed and intravenous abciximab infusion (0.125 μg/kg/min) was initiated. (*C*) The aneurysm was then coiled to near-complete occlusion. The patient emerged from general anesthesia neurologically intact and was administered loading doses of aspirin and clopidogrel.

represents a critical component of therapy, because up to 50% of subjects exhibit subtherapeutic platelet inhibition after a weight-based dose of a IIb/IIIa inhibitor [40].

Some have argued for a continuous heparin drip after neuroendovascular stenting procedures. All investigations of this strategy in the coronary literature have indicated little efficacy in preventing thrombotic complications with significant cost with respect to incidence of hemorrhagic events, however [66,67].

After a stent has been placed, dual-antiplatelet therapy is required for a minimum of 4 to 6 weeks. When a stent has been placed for aneurysm embolization in a large (>3.5 mm) intracranial

vessel, we typically maintain patients on aspirin (162–325 mg) and clopidogrel (75 mg) for 6 weeks, with aspirin to be continued indefinitely thereafter. If a stent (carotid or intracranial) is placed for atherostenosis, the existing literature suggests that continued treatment with aspirin (162–325 mg/d) and clopidogrel (75 mg/d) may be beneficial for as long as 1 year [21].

Management of intraprocedural thromboembolic complications

Thromboembolic events account for most of the complications related to the endovascular treatment of intracranial lesions. Advancing the

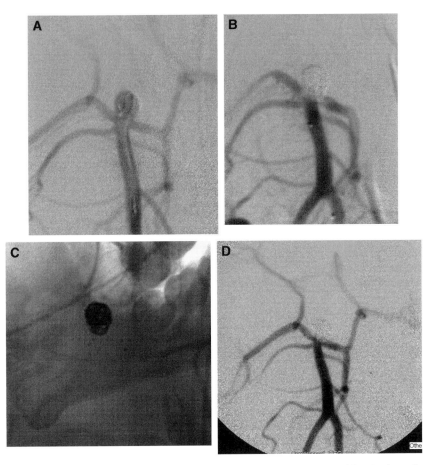

Fig. 4. A 22-year-old woman with an unruptured basilar artery apex aneurysm presented for elective coil embolization. (*A*) A three-dimensional coil produced adequate framing of the aneurysm. Subsequent coil embolization was performed with increasing occlusion of the aneurysm. (*B*) As additional coils were introduced into the aneurysm, however, the three-dimensional coil began to protrude slightly into the basilar apex and thrombus began to accumulate within the basilar apex and extend into the proximal posterior cerebral arteries. Abciximab (10 mg) was administered intra-arterially through a microcatheter positioned just proximal to the basilar apex. (*C*) Subsequently, a 4.5-mm × 15-mm Neuroform stent was placed, extending from the P1 segment of the posterior cerebral artery (PCA) proximally into the distal third of the basilar artery. Follow-up angiography demonstrated complete resolution of the thrombus and restoration of patency to the basilar apex and PCA. The remainder of the abciximab bolus was administered through a peripheral intravenous line. Because the aneurysm was unruptured, 12-hour abciximab infusion was administered. The patient emerged from general anesthesia neurologically intact and was loaded with aspirin and clopidogrel.

ability to prevent, identify, and manage such complications is one of the most efficacious ways by which to optimize the risk-benefit ratio of endovascular therapy.

Most operators fully heparinize patients during endovascular intervention to reduce the incidence of thromboembolic complications. In the setting of an acutely hemorrhagic index lesion, some operators delay full intraprocedural anticoagulation until the lesion is partially secured. Workman et al [68] proposed the strategy of pretreating patients with antiplatelet agents

(aspirin alone or aspirin with clopidogrel) to reduce the risk of thromboembolism during the treatment of unruptured aneurysms even further. Despite these preventative measures, angiographically perceptible thromboembolic complications have been reported to occur with a frequency of 6.7% [68].

Thromboembolic complications encountered during the endovascular treatment of hemorrhagic or potentially hemorrhagic vascular lesions represent a particularly challenging problem. The operator must determine the most effective means by which to achieve clot dissolution without provoking hemorrhage from the target lesion.

Two classes of pharmacologic agents have been applied in this situation—thrombolytic agents (eg, tissue plasminogen activator [tPA] and urokinase) and GP IIb/IIIa inhibitors. Recombinant tissue plasminogen activator (rtPA; eg, alteplase) acts by converting plasminogen to plasmin. Plasmin is also an active serine protease that acts primarily to lyse fibrin and thereby produce thrombolysis. The efficiency of tPA-mediated plasminogen activation is markedly enhanced in the presence of fibrin, which provides a surface for the sequential binding of tPA and plasminogen. By acting primarily on fibrin-entrapped plasminogen, tPA has a more specific localized thrombolytic effect, with less of an associated systemic fibrinolytic action. Cronqvist et al [69] reported the use of urokinase to manage intra- and periprocedural thromboembolic complications encountered during GDC embolization in 19 patients. The investigators reported excellent angiographic results, with partial or complete recanalization achieved in all cases, as well as a good clinical outcome in 74% of patients. Only 6 patients in the series had acutely ruptured aneurysms, however, and in this subset, 3 patients experienced significant hemorrhagic complications after thrombolysis. Koebbe et al [70] used thrombolytic agents to manage thromboembolic complications in a series of 5 patients undergoing embolization of aneurysms. Two of the 5 experienced fatal subarachnoid hemorrhage after thrombolysis. One of these patients had a previously unruptured aneurysm. Taken together, the available data indicate that thrombolytic agents, although effective in achieving dissolution of intraprocedural thrombi, are probably associated with an approximately 50% rate of symptomatic and, in many cases, fatal intracranial hemorrhage when used in the setting of an acutely hemorrhagic aneurysm.

Hyperacute thromboemboli identified during the course of neuroendovascular procedures likely represent primarily aggregates of activated platelets that are not yet stabilized by fibrin cross-linking. For this reason, the GP IIb/IIIa inhibitors, which block the final common pathway of platelet aggregation, are uniquely suited to prevent propagation of hyperacute thrombi without disrupting more subacute fibrin-stabilized thrombi, which stabilize acutely or subacutely hemorrhagic vascular lesions. To date, the use of GP IIb/IIIa inhibitors for the management of intraprocedural thromboembolic events has been documented in 54 patients (22 intravenous and 32 intra-arterial, with 52 patients with hemorrhagic or potentially hemorrhagic vascular lesions), with complete or partial resolution of thrombus in 52 of 54 cases and no documented cases of new or increased intracranial hemorrhage related to the index lesion (Table 1).

In our experience, intra-arterial and intravenous abciximab are effective. The intra-arterial route of administration has two major advantages: the instantaneous achievement of high local concentrations of the drug with a rapid onset of action and the fact that adequate thrombolysis may be achieved at a lower total dose. In our experience [71], the intra-arterial route of administration results in a faster rate of clot dissolution (<5 minutes), whereas the intravenous route of administration requires more time (>10 minutes). We have administered abciximab intra-arterially at up to 0.25 mg/kg (the recommended loading dose). We administer the intra-arterial dose in

Table 1
Summary of available case series reporting the administration of glycoprotein IIb/IIIa inhibitors for the management of thromboembolic complications encountered during endovascular procedures

Study (reference number)	Number of patients	IIB/IIIA agent (route of administration, number of patients)
Wallace et al, 1997 [93]	1	Abciximab (IV)
Lempert et al, 1999 [94]	1	Abciximab (IV)
Tong et al, 2000 [95]	1	Abciximab (IV)
Cloft et al, 2001 [96]	4	Abciximab (IV)
Ng et al, 2001 [97]	1	Abciximab (IV)
Duncan et al, 2002 [98]	5	Abciximab (IA)
Kwon et al, 2002 [99]	2	Abciximab (IA)
Alexander et al, 2002 [100]	1	Abciximab (IV)
Workman et al, 2002 [68]	5	Abciximab (IV, 4); Eptifibatide (IV, 1)
Fiorella et al, 2004 [71]	13	Abciximab (IV, 8; IA, 5)
Mounayer et al, 2003 [101]	13	Abciximab (IA 13) 4 ruptured
Song et al, 2004 [102]	7	Abciximab (IA 7) 4 ruptured

Abbreviations: IA, intra-arterial; IV, intravenous.

2- to 5-mg aliquots through a microcatheter positioned in the vicinity of the thrombus and perform control angiography periodically through the guiding catheter to document the status of the clot. Additional doses are administered intra-arterially as needed to achieve adequate thrombolysis. Adequate lysis is sometimes achieved after the first or second aliquot administered (see Fig. 4). Correspondingly, the intra-arterial administration of abciximab using this methodology results in a lower total dose of abciximab than that administered by the intravenous route, in which the entire dose (0.25 mg/kg) is administered as a bolus. The lower dose of abciximab used with this technique of intra-arterial administration should be associated with a shorter and less intense inhibition of systemic platelet function. Correspondingly, intra-arterial administration would be expected to involve a lower risk of intra- and extracranial hemorrhagic complications.

If the thromboembolic complication occurred as a sequela of a permanent thrombogenic foreign body (eg, a coil pack with some extension into the parent vessel) implanted in the setting of an acutely hemorrhagic lesion (eg, ruptured aneurysm or AVM), the patient is started on aspirin (162–325 mg) immediately after the procedure, provided that no hemorrhagic complication is identified on postprocedural CT imaging. In these cases, antiplatelet therapy (aspirin at a dose of 81 mg/d) is continued indefinitely unless discontinuation is required for another interventional procedure (eg, ventriculoperitoneal shunt placement). Because most thromboembolic complications related to aneurysm embolization occur within the first 24 to 48 hours, it is best if such procedures can be delayed for at least 2 days after the initial procedure [72].

The intravenous route of administration as a bolus and infusion provides a longer duration of platelet blockade and does not require the super-selective positioning of a microcatheter. If a thromboembolic complication occurs as the result of a fixed intravascular thrombogenic focus implanted during the treatment of a lesion that has not recently hemorrhaged, a longer acting platelet blockade may be advantageous. In these situations, the thrombus is also frequently small (seen as a filling defect adherent to the coil pack) and does not compromise flow within the parent vessel. Correspondingly, the slightly slower onset of action observed with the intravenous route of abciximab administration is also usually acceptable in these situations. The intravenous route of administration is technically easier and may also be optimal for thromboembolic complications observed during diagnostic angiography, in which the introduction and selective positioning of a microcatheter would entail a significant delay in therapy.

Acute stroke intervention

At the time of percutaneous intervention, most thromboembolic occlusions are caused primarily by relatively organized clot containing platelets, thrombin, and fibrin mesh. After successful fibrinolysis with an agent like rtPA, thrombin and other soluble agonists are released locally in high concentrations, resulting in local platelet activation and aggregation. Aggregation of these activated platelets may obstruct the distal microcirculation and frequently result in reocclusion at the point of the initial obstruction [73–75]. In addition, the new thrombus generated is predominantly composed of platelets and is thus relatively resistant to the effects of the fibrinolytic agents. This phenomenon is observed not only in the cerebrovasculature but in the coronary circulation. For this reason, interventional cardiologists began to use abciximab in concert with fibrinolytic agents to facilitate recanalization of occluded coronary arteries. In the Thrombolysis in Myocardial Infarction (TIMI) [76] 14 study (888 patients), the addition of abciximab augmented the rate and extent of thrombolysis with reduced doses of alteplase. TIMI grade 3 flow at 60 minutes increased from 43% with alteplase alone to 72% using a 50 mg regimen of alteplase over 60 minutes combined with abciximab—a 67% relative increase and a 29% absolute difference in TIMI grade 3 flow rates. Ohman et al [77] observed a similar benefit when eptifibatide was combined with alteplase in patients undergoing acute MI with more complete reperfusion (TIMI grade 3 flow, 66% versus 39%) and a shorter median time to ST-segment recovery in those patients receiving eptifibatide.

Little data exist describing the efficacy of IIb/IIIa inhibitors for the treatment of acute stroke. The combination of IIb/IIIa inhibitors with rtPA significantly reduced infarct size and improved neurologic outcome in a rat model of embolic stroke [78]. In a rabbit stroke model, animals given IIb/IIIa inhibitor with rtPA also paradoxically showed significantly fewer intracerebral hemorrhages than those given rtPA alone [79].

The investigators theorized that the increased rate of hemorrhage in the rtPA-only group may have been attributable to increased reocclusion of cerebral vessels after initial thrombolysis.

In an acute ischemic stroke study, abciximab was administered parenterally to 54 stroke patients up to 24 hours (median of 12 hours) after the onset of symptoms. Although this therapy resulted in 10 asymptomatic cerebral hemorrhages in the abciximab group compared with only 1 in the placebo group, the number of symptomatic hemorrhages did not increase and the abciximab group trended toward a higher rate of excellent recovery at 3 months compared with the placebo group [80]. Seitz et al [81] compared intravenous rtPA with intravenous rtPA plus tirofiban. The patients who received rtPA and IIb/IIIa inhibitors had no higher incidence of hemorrhagic conversion and also had a better modified Rankin Scale (mRS) score at discharge compared with controls. Eckert et al [82] treated 3 patients with vertebrobasilar occlusion with local intra-arterial rtPA in combination with abciximab. Recanalization with clinical improvement occurred in 2 of the 3 patients, and there were no hemorrhagic complications. Junghans et al [83] treated 18 patients with progressive acute ischemic stroke with intravenous tirofiban. None of the patients suffered a major intracranial hemorrhage, and 6 patients sustained asymptomatic hemorrhagic conversion of their stroke.

Although the application of IIb/IIIa inhibitors to achieve acute revascularization likely represents a safe and efficacious strategy, caution must be exercised in those patients already treated with antiplatelet agents. Cheung and Ho [84] reported massive hemorrhagic transformation of an ischemic cerebral infarction in a patient given intravenous abciximab who had been on aspirin and Ticlid therapy. Qureshi et al [62] reported seven patients who developed fatal intracerebral hemorrhages after receiving abciximab during neurointerventional procedures. In all seven patients, abciximab was used in combination with heparin and clopidogrel.

We have recently completed a study designed to examine the safety of the combined administration of intra-arterial rtPA and IIb/IIIa inhibitors in the setting of acute stroke [85]. In our case series, we sought to use primarily rtPA and mechanical thrombolysis with compliant balloon angioplasty to achieve flow restoration. Subsequent intra-arterial IIb/IIIa administration was undertaken only in cases in which attempted rtPA and/or mechanical thrombolysis primarily failed or in the setting of acute reocclusion after initially successful thrombolysis. Of the 21 patients who received combined therapy, 3 patients had asymptomatic postprocedural hemorrhages on CT. No symptomatic or fatal hemorrhagic complications were observed. Partial or complete recanalization occurred in 17 of 21 patients (81%) despite the selection of failed cases. After thrombolysis, 62% of patients were functionally independent (mRS score of 0–3), including half of those patients who presented with basilar thrombosis. These results compare favorably with those of the Prolyse in Acute Cerebral Thromboembolism II (PROACT II) study [86], which documented a recanalization rate of 66% and a rate of intracerebral hemorrhage associated with neurologic deterioration of 10% within 24 hours. A more relevant comparison can be made to case series in which salvage angioplasty was pursued in the patients resistant to thrombolytic infusion. Ringer et al [87] reported a recanalization rate of 56% in 9 patients with inadequate recanalization after initial thrombolytic infusion. Ueda et al [88] performed balloon angioplasty in acute stroke patients with more than 70% stenosis of the offending vessel after thrombolysis. Their recanalization rate was 84% in 13 patients; however, not all the patients had an occlusion refractory to local thrombolytics.

On the basis of these results, we have started to incorporate abciximab into our routine armamentarium for the treatment of acute stroke in those cases in which the US Food and Drug Administration–approved mechanisms for clot retrieval are not possible or do not yield sufficient recanalization. In these instances, we administer alternating doses of rtPA and abciximab in concert with compliant balloon angioplasty to achieve primary recanalization. On the basis of our previous experience, we limit our doses of abciximab to 0.125 mg/kg (one half of the recommended intravenous loading bolus). In these cases, we are not attempting to achieve a systemic level of therapeutic inhibition of platelet activity; as such, we do not routinely verify platelet inhibition with platelet function testing.

Stroke prevention

With increasing frequency, the interventional neuroradiologist and endovascular neurosurgeon are involved in determining appropriate treatment regimens for stroke prevention in patients with symptomatic carotid and intracranial atheromatous disease. As such, the question arises as to the optimal preventative therapy for acute stroke in these patients. This topic remains the subject of avid contention, and no widely accepted conclusion has been reached at this point.

When evaluating the available data, it is important to consider that most patients evaluated by the neurointerventionist represent only a fraction of the overall cohort of patients requiring pharmacotherapy for secondary prevention for stroke. Only 20% of ischemic stroke is accounted for by patients with atherosclerotic cerebrovascular disease, whereas the remainder is composed of patients with penetrating artery disease and/or small-vessel ischemic disease (25%), cardiogenic embolic disease (20%), cryptogenic causes (30%), and other more rare causes (5%; hypercoagulable states, dissection, vasculitis, vasospasm, and drug related). The heterogeneity of this disease process is particularly relevant in the acute postinfarct period, in which patients with large-artery atheromatous disease are at a much greater risk of clinical deterioration and recurrent stroke. The 30-day risk of recurrent stroke has been reported to be approximately 8% for these patients, which is six times greater than that observed in patients with nonatheromatous stroke [89,90].

As such, much of the available data from the preventative neurology literature (which groups all patients together) is not directly applicable to neuroendovascular patients. Arguably, the subset of the disease process treated by the neuroendovascular interventionist (intra- and extracranial large-vessel atheromatous disease) is more analogous to symptomatic CAD than it is to the remainder of the ischemic stroke population. Correspondingly, it is probably prudent to take guidance from the preventative cardiology literature as well as from the "all-inclusive" preventative stroke literature.

For symptomatic patients who have not been previously treated with an antiplatelet agent, single antiplatelet therapy is probably adequate, consisting of aspirin (50–325 mg/d) or clopidogrel (75 mg/d). Data from the CAPRIE trial [15] and the Ticlopidine Aspirin Stroke Study Group [91] would suggest that there may be a small benefit in choosing a thienopyridine over aspirin as a single agent from the standpoint of the prevention of vascular events as well as from that of a lower risk of a bleeding complication. The only compelling reasons to choose clopidogrel as a first-line agent are aspirin intolerance or aspirin resistance as demonstrated by platelet aggregation studies. Whether there is a beneficial effect of adding clopidogrel to aspirin for stroke prevention is not currently known. Although the CURE study [51] suggests a benefit of dual therapy for the prevention of vascular events, the MATCH study results argue against this.

A recent meta-analysis (merged data from 7 trials involving 11,459 patients) supported the utility of extended-release dipyridamole in addition to aspirin for secondary stroke prevention, with the combination of agents yielding a significant benefit when compared with aspirin therapy alone in patients with previous ischemic stroke or TIA (22% RRR when compared with aspirin alone and 39% RRR in comparison to placebo). Although much of the data supporting the utility of dipyridamole was derived from a single study, ESPS-II, a significant benefit was still observed when these data were excluded from the meta-analysis [92]. Significantly less data exist supporting the utility of dipyridamole in comparison to the other antiplatelet agents, however, and further study is warranted. Two large trials are now underway that should provide further insight into this issue: the ESPRIT (anticoagulation versus aspirin at a dose of 30–325 mg/d versus aspirin at a dose of 20 mg) with extended-release dipyridamole (200 mg administered twice a day), and the Prevention Regimen for Effectively Avoiding Secondary Strokes (PRoFESS) (aspirin with extended-release dipyridamole versus clopidogrel). Given the relative paucity of data directly evaluating the efficacy of dipyridamole in the population of patients with large-vessel atheromatous disease and the theoretic risk of exacerbating coronary artery ischemia in patients with significant CAD, we prefer aspirin or clopidogrel as a primary agent for stroke prevention pending the results of the trials that are currently underway.

Regardless of the agent selected, as they become more widely available, platelet function tests should provide a useful means by which to verify the efficacy of the chosen therapy. If a given regimen produces inadequate levels of platelet inhibition, the dosing regimens or agents used should be changed. Also, if aspirin is used as the agent of choice, periodic platelet function tests may be indicated, because previous studies have demonstrated that resistance to aspirin therapy may develop over time [9]. Platelet function should always be assessed with any evidence of treatment failure so as to verify the continued efficacy of the agent used and to evaluate patient compliance.

If a patient fails single-agent therapy with aspirin as indicated by a neurologic or nonneurologic vascular event (MI or peripheral vascular event), the patient should be changed to clopidogrel or clopidogrel should be added to the aspirin therapy [29]. If the patient fails adequate dual-antiplatelet therapy, neuroendovascular intervention or cerebrovascular bypass options should be strongly considered. If revascularization procedures are not feasible, the addition of coumadin should be considered.

Summary

Our understanding of the pharmacology of antiplatelet therapy continues to evolve rapidly. Although the existing data are primarily generated in the setting of interventional and preventative cardiology studies, these data may be extrapolated to guide the rational application of these agents in neuroendovascular procedures. Platelet function testing represents an increasingly available and practical method by which to verify the adequacy of therapy and guide clinical decision making. The optimal application of these agents will undoubtedly improve the risk profile of neuroendovascular procedures, increase the success rate of acute stroke intervention, and facilitate more effective secondary stroke prevention.

References

[1] Baier RE, Dutton RC. Initial events in interactions of blood with a foreign surface. J Biomed Mater Res 1969;3:191–206.

[2] Schafer AI. Anti-platelet therapy. Am J Med 1996; 101:199–209.

[3] Taylor DW, Barnett HJ, Haynes RB, et al. Low-dose and high-dose acetylsalicylic acid for patients undergoing carotid endarterectomy: a randomised controlled trial. ASA and Carotid Endarterectomy (ACE) Trial Collaborators. Lancet 1999;353(9171): 2179–84.

[4] Patrono C. Aspirin as an antiplatelet drug. N Engl J Med 1994;330:1287–94.

[5] Awtry EH, Loscalzo J. Aspirin. Circulation 2000; 101:1206–18.

[6] Gum PA, Kottke-Marchant K, Welsh PA, et al. A prospective, blinded determination of the natural history of aspirin resistance among stable patients with cardiovascular disease. J Am Coll Cardiol 2003;41(6):961–5.

[7] Chen WH, Lee PY, Ng W, et al. Aspirin resistance is associated with a high incidence of myonecrosis after non-urgent percutaneous coronary intervention despite clopidogrel pretreatment. J Am Coll Cardiol 2004;43(6):1122–6.

[8] Alberts MJ, Bergman DL, Molner E, et al. Antiplatelet effect of aspirin in patients with cerebrovascular disease. Stroke 2004;35:175–8.

[9] Pulcinelli FM, Pignatelli P, Celestini A, et al. Inhibition of platelet aggregation by aspirin progressively decreases in long-term treated patients. J Am Coll Cardiol 2004;43(6):979–84.

[10] Grotemeyer KH, Scharafinski HW, Husstedt IW. Two-year follow-up of aspirin responders and aspirin non responders: a pilot-study including 180 post-stroke patients. Thromb Res 1993;71: 397–403.

[11] Mueller MR, Salat A, Stangl P, et al. Variable platelet response to low-dose ASA and the risk of limb deterioration in patients submitted to peripheral arterial angioplasty. Thromb Haemost 1997; 78(3):1003–7.

[12] Quinn MJ, Fitzgerald DJ. Ticlopidine and clopidogrel. Circulation 1999;100:1667–72.

[13] Bertrand ME, Rupprecht HJ, Urban P, et al. Double-blind study of the safety of clopidogrel with and without a loading dose in combination with aspirin compared with ticlopidine in combination with aspirin after coronary stenting: the Clopidogrel Aspirin Stent International Cooperative Study (CLASSICS). Circulation 2000;102(6): 624–9.

[14] Muller I, Seyfarth M, Rudiger S, et al. Effect of a high loading dose of clopidogrel on platelet function in patients undergoing coronary stent placement. Heart 2001;85(1):92–3.

[15] CAPRIE Steering Committee. A randomised, blinded, trial of clopidogrel versus aspirin in patients at risk of ischaemic events (CAPRIE). Lancet 1996;348(9038):1329–39.

[16] Patrono C, Bachmann F, Baigent C, et al. Expert consensus document on the use of antiplatelet agents. The task force on the use of antiplatelet agents in patients with atherosclerotic cardiovascular disease of the European Society of Cardiology. Eur Heart J 2004;25(2):166–81.

[17] Savcic M, Hauert J, Bachmann F, et al. Clopidogrel loading dose regimens: kinetic profile of pharmacodynamic response in healthy subjects. Semin Thromb Hemost 1999;25(Suppl 2):15–9.

[18] Gurbel PA, Cummings CC, Bell CR, et al. Plavix Reduction of New Thrombus Occurrence (PRONTO) trial. Onset and extent of platelet inhibition by clopidogrel loading in patients undergoing elective coronary stenting: the Plavix Reduction of New Thrombus Occurrence (PRONTO) trial. Am Heart J 2003;145(2):239–47.

[19] Cadroy Y, Bossavy JP, Thalamas C, et al. Early potent antithrombotic effect with combined aspirin and a loading dose of clopidogrel on experimental arterial thrombogenesis in humans. Circulation 2000;101(24):2823–8.

[20] Patrono C. Pharmacology of antiplatelet agents. In: Loscalzo J, Schafer AI, editors. Thrombosis and hemorrhage. Baltimore: William & Wilkins; 1998. p. 261–91.

[21] Steinhubl SR, Berger PB, Mann JT III, et al. Early and sustained dual oral antiplatelet therapy following percutaneous coronary intervention: a randomized controlled trial. JAMA 2002;288:2411–20.

[22] Gurbel PA, Bliden KP, Hiatt BL, et al. Clopidogrel for coronary stenting: response variability, drug resistance, and the effect of pretreatment platelet reactivity. Circulation 2003;107(23):2908–13.

[23] Muller I, Besta F, Schulz C, et al. Prevalence of clopidogrel non-responders among patients with stable angina pectoris scheduled for elective coronary stent placement. Thromb Haemost 2003;89(5):783–7.

[24] Lau WC, Gurbel PA, Watkins PB, et al. Contribution of hepatic cytochrome P450 3A4 metabolic activity to the phenomenon of clopidogrel resistance. Circulation 2004;109(2):166–71.

[25] Matetzky S, Shenkman B, Guetta V, et al. Clopidogrel resistance is associated with increased risk of recurrent atherothrombotic events in patients with acute myocardial infarction. Circulation 2004;109(25):3171–5.

[26] Gurbel PA, Bliden KP. Durability of platelet inhibition by clopidogrel. Am J Cardiol 2003;91(9): 1123–5.

[27] Fitzgerald GA. Dipyridamole. N Engl J Med 1987; 316(20):1247–57.

[28] Diener HC, Cunha L, Forbes C, et al. European Stroke Prevention Study. 2. Dipyridamole and acetylsalicylic acid in the secondary prevention of stroke. J Neurol Sci 1996;143(1–2):1–13.

[29] Tran H, Anand SS. Oral antiplatelet therapy in cerebrovascular disease, coronary artery disease, and peripheral arterial disease. JAMA 2004;292(15): 1867–74.

[30] Coller BS. Platelet GPIIb/IIIa antagonists: the first anti-integrin receptor therapeutics. J Clin Invest 1997;99(7):1467–71.

[31] Gawaz M, Neumann FJ, Schomig A. Evaluation of platelet membrane glycoproteins in coronary artery disease: consequences for diagnosis and therapy. Circulation 1999;99(1):E1–11.

[32] Tcheng JE, Talley JD, O'Shea JC, et al. Clinical pharmacology of higher dose eptifibatide in percutaneous coronary intervention (the PRIDE study). Am J Cardiol 2001;88:1097–102.

[33] ESPRIT Investigators. Enhanced suppression of the platelet IIb/IIIa receptor with Integrilin therapy. Novel dosing regimen of eptifibatide in planned coronary stent implantation (ESPRIT): a randomised, placebo-controlled trial. Lancet 2000;356(9247):2037–44.

[34] RESTORE Investigators. Effects of platelet glycoprotein IIb/IIIa blockade with tirofiban on adverse cardiac events in patients with unstable angina or acute myocardial infarction undergoing coronary angioplasty. The RESTORE Investigators. Randomized Efficacy Study of Tirofiban for Outcomes and REstenosis. Circulation 1997; 96(5):1445–53.

[35] Smith SC Jr, Dove JT, Jacobs AK, et al. ACC/ AHA guidelines for percutaneous coronary intervention. Circulation 2001;103(24):3019–41.

[36] The EPILOG Investigators. Platelet glycoprotein IIb/IIIa receptor blockade and low-dose heparin during percutaneous coronary revascularization. N Engl J Med 1997;336(24):1689–96.

[37] Neumann FJ, Hochholzer W, Pogatsa-Murray G, et al. Antiplatelet effects of abciximab, tirofiban and eptifibatide in patients undergoing coronary stenting. J Am Coll Cardiol 2001;37(5): 1323–8.

[38] Kleiman NS, Raizner AE, Jordan R, et al. Differential inhibition of platelet aggregation induced by adenosine diphosphate or a thrombin receptor-activating peptide in patients treated with bolus chimeric 7E3 Fab: implications for inhibition of the internal pool of GPIIb/IIIa receptors. J Am Coll Cardiol 1995;26(7):1665–71.

[39] Renda G, Rocca B, Crocchiolo R, et al. Effect of fibrinogen concentration and platelet count on the inhibitory effect of abciximab and tirofiban. Thromb Haemost 2003;89(2):348–54.

[40] Kini AS, Richard M, Suleman J, et al. Effectiveness of tirofiban, eptifibatide, and abciximab in minimizing myocardial necrosis during percutaneous coronary intervention (TEAM pilot study). Am J Cardiol 2002;90(5):526–9.

[41] Steinhubl SR, Talley JD, Braden GA, et al. Point-of-care measured platelet inhibition correlates with a reduced risk of an adverse cardiac event after percutaneous coronary intervention: results of the GOLD (AU-Assessing Ultegra) multicenter study. Circulation 2001;103(21):2572–8.

[42] Li YF, Spencer FA, Becker RC. Comparative efficacy of fibrinogen and platelet supplementation on the in vitro reversibility of competitive glycoprotein IIb/IIIa receptor-directed platelet inhibition. Am Heart J 2002;143(4):725–32.

[43] Topol EJ, Moliterno DJ, Herrmann HC, et al. TARGET Investigators. Do Tirofiban and ReoPro Give Similar Efficacy Trial. Comparison of two platelet glycoprotein IIb/IIIa inhibitors, tirofiban and abciximab, for the prevention of ischemic events with percutaneous coronary revascularization. N Engl J Med 2001;344(25): 1888–94.

[44] Burns ER, Lawrence C. Bleeding time. A guide to its diagnostic and clinical utility. Arch Pathol Lab Med 1989;113:1219–24.

[45] Proimos G. Platelet aggregation inhibition with glycoprotein IIb-IIIa inhibitors. J Thromb Thrombolysis 2001;11(2):99–110.

[46] Harrington RA, Kleiman NS, Kottke-Marchant K, et al. Immediate and reversible platelet inhibition after intravenous administration of a peptide glycoprotein IIb/IIIa inhibitor during percutaneous coronary intervention. Am J Cardiol 1995;76(17):1222–7.

[47] VerifyNow™ package insert reference: VerifyNow™ Aspirin Improved [package insert]. San Diego, CA: Accumetrics Inc; 2004.

[48] Antithrombotic Trialists' Collaboration. Collaborative meta-analysis of randomised trials of antiplatelet therapy for prevention of death, myocardial infarction, and stroke in high risk patients. BMJ 2002;324(7329):71–86.

[49] Bhatt DL, Hirsch AT, Ringleb PA, et al. Reduction in the need for hospitalization for recurrent ischemic events and bleeding with clopidogrel instead of aspirin. CAPRIE Investigators. Am Heart J 2000;140(1):67–73.

[50] Bassavy JP, Thomas C, Sagnard L, et al. A double-blind randomized comparison of combined aspirin and ticlopidine therapy versus aspirin or ticlopidine alone on experimental arterial thrombogenesis in humans. Blood 1998;92(5):1518–25.

[51] Peters RJ, Mehta SR, Fox KA, et al. Clopidogrel in Unstable angina to prevent Recurrent Events (CURE) Trial Investigators. Effects of aspirin dose when used alone or in combination with clopidogrel in patients with acute coronary syndromes: observations from the Clopidogrel in Unstable angina to prevent Recurrent Events (CURE) study. Circulation 2003;108(14):1682–7.

[52] Mehta SR, Yusuf S, Peters RJ, et al. Clopidogrel in Unstable angina to prevent Recurrent Events trial (CURE) Investigators. Effects of pretreatment with clopidogrel and aspirin followed by long-term therapy in patients undergoing percutaneous coronary intervention: the PCI-CURE study. Lancet 2001;358(9281):527–33.

[53] Rozenman Y. For how long should treatment with clopidogrel be continued after coronary stent implantation? J Am Coll Cardiol 2004;43(7):1331–2.

[54] Diener HC, Bogousslavsky J, Brass LM, et al. MATCH Investigators Aspirin and clopidogrel compared with clopidogrel alone after recent ischaemic stroke or transient ischaemic attack in high-risk patients (MATCH): randomised, double-blind, placebo-controlled trial. Lancet 2004;24;364(9431):331–7.

[55] Kastrati A, Mehilli J, Schuhlen H, et al. Intracoronary Stenting and Antithrombotic Regimen-Rapid Early Action for Coronary Treatment Study Investigators. A clinical trial of abciximab in elective percutaneous coronary intervention after pretreatment with clopidogrel. N Engl J Med 2004;350(3):232–8.

[56] The EPIC Investigators. Use of a monoclonal antibody directed against the platelet glycoprotein IIb/IIIa receptor in high-risk coronary angioplasty. N Engl J Med 1994;330(14):956–61.

[57] Klootwijk P, Meij S, Melkert R, et al. Reduction of recurrent ischemia with abciximab during continuous ECG-ischemia monitoring in patients with unstable angina refractory to standard treatment (CAPTURE). Circulation 1998;98(14):1358–64.

[58] The EPISTENT Investigators. Randomised placebo-controlled and balloon-angioplasty-controlled trial to assess safety of coronary stenting with use of platelet glycoprotein-IIb/IIIa blockade. Lancet 1998;352(9122):87–92.

[59] Topol EJ, Mark DB, Lincoff AM, et al. Outcomes at 1 year and economic implications of platelet glycoprotein IIb/IIIa blockade in patients undergoing coronary stenting: results from a multicentre randomised trial. Lancet 1999;354(9195):2019–24.

[60] The IMPACT-II Investigators. Randomised placebo-controlled trial of effect of eptifibatide on complications of percutaneous coronary intervention: IMPACT-II. Lancet 1997;349(9063):1422–8.

[61] The RESTORE Investigators. Effects of platelet glycoprotein IIb/IIIa blockade with tirofiban on adverse cardiac events in patients with unstable angina or acute myocardial infarction undergoing coronary angioplasty. Circulation 1997;96(5):1445–53.

[62] Qureshi AI, Saad M, Zaidat OO, et al. Intracerebral hemorrhages associated with neurointerventional procedures using a combination of antithrombotic agents including abciximab. Stroke 2002;33(7):1916–9.

[63] Qureshi AI, Suri MF, Ali Z, et al. Carotid angioplasty and stent placement: a prospective analysis of perioperative complications and impact of intravenously administered abciximab. Neurosurgery 2002;50(3):466–73.

[64] Al Siddiqui AM, Hanel RA, Xavier AR, et al. Safety of high-dose intravenous eptifibatide as an adjunct to internal carotid artery angioplasty and stent placement: a prospective registry. Neurosurgery 2004;54(2):307–16.

[65] Qureshi AI, Ali Z, Suri MF, et al. Open-label phase I clinical study to assess the safety of intravenous eptifibatide in patients undergoing internal carotid artery angioplasty and stent placement. Neurosurgery 2001;48(5):998–1004.

[66] Ellis SG, Roubin GS, Wilentz J, et al. Effect of 18- to 24-hour heparin administration for prevention of restenosis after uncomplicated coronary angioplasty. Am Heart J 1989;117(4):777–82.

[67] Friedman HZ, Cragg DR, Glazier SM, et al. Randomized prospective evaluation of prolonged versus abbreviated intravenous heparin therapy after coronary angioplasty. J Am Coll Cardiol 1994;24(5):1214–9.

[68] Workman MJ, Cloft HJ, Tong FC, et al. Thrombus formation at the neck of cerebral aneurysms during

treatment with Guglielmi detachable coils. AJNR Am J Neuroradiol 2002;23(9):1568–76.

[69] Cronqvist M, Pierot L, Boulin A, et al. Local intra-arterial fibrinolysis of thromboemboli occurring during endovascular treatment of intracerebral aneurysm: a comparison of anatomic results and clinical outcome. AJNR Am J Neuroradiol 1998; 19(1):157–65.

[70] Koebbe CJ, Horowitz MB, Levy EI, et al. Intra-arterial thrombolysis for thromboemboli associated with endovascular aneurysm coiling. Report of five cases. Intervent Neuroradiol 2002;8:151–8.

[71] Fiorella D, Albuquerque FC, Han P, et al. Strategies for the management of intraprocedural thromboembolic complications with abciximab (ReoPro). Neurosurgery 2004;54(5):1089–97.

[72] Derdeyn CP, Cross DT III, Moran CJ, et al. Post-procedure ischemic events after treatment of intra-cranial aneurysms with Guglielmi detachable coils. J Neurosurg 2000;96(5):837–43.

[73] Fitzgerald DJ, Catella F, Roy L, et al. Marked platelet activation in vivo after intravenous strepto-kinase in patients with acute myocardial infarction. Circulation 1988;77(1):142–50.

[74] Owen J, Friedman KD, Grossmann BA, et al. Thrombolytic therapy with tissue-plasminogen activator or streptokinase induces transient thrombin activity. Blood 1988;72(2):616–20.

[75] Merlini PA, Bauer KA, Oltrona L, et al. Thrombin generation and activity during thrombolysis and concomitant heparin therapy in patients with acute myocardial infarction. J Am Coll Cardiol 1995; 25(1):203–9.

[76] Antman EM, Giugliano RP, Gibson CM, et al. Abciximab facilitates the rate and extent of throm-bolysis: results of the Thrombolysis in Myocardial Infarction (TIMI) 14 trial. The TIMI 14 Investiga-tors. Circulation 1999;99(21):2720–32.

[77] Ohman EM, Kleiman NS, Gacioch G, et al. Com-bined accelerated tissue-plasminogen activator and platelet glycoprotein IIb/IIIa integrin receptor blockade with Integrilin in acute myocardial infarc-tion. Results of a randomized, placebo-controlled, dose-ranging trial. IMPACT-AMI Investigators. Circulation 1997;95(4):846–54.

[78] Zhang L, Zhang ZG, Zhang R, et al. Adjuvant treatment with a glycoprotein IIb/IIIa receptor in-hibitor increases the therapeutic window for low-dose tissue plasminogen activator administration in a rat model of embolic stroke. Circulation 2003;107(22):2837–43.

[79] Lapchak PA, Araujo DM, Song D, et al. The non-peptide glycoprotein IIb/IIIa platelet receptor an-tagonist SM-20302 reduces tissue plasminogen activator-induced intracerebral hemorrhage after thromboembolic stroke. Stroke 2002;33(1):147–52.

[80] Abciximab in Ischemic Stroke Investigators. Abciximab in acute ischemic stroke: a randomized,

double-blind, placebo-controlled, dose-escalation study. Stroke 2000;31(3):601–9.

[81] Seitz RJ, Hamzavi M, Junghans U, et al. Throm-bolysis with recombinant tissue plasminogen activator and tirofiban in stroke: preliminary observations. Stroke 2003;34(8):1932–5.

[82] Eckert B, Koch C, Thomalla G, et al. Acute basilar artery occlusion treated with combined intravenous abciximab and intra-arterial tissue plasminogen activator: report of 3 cases. Stroke 2002;33(5):1424–7.

[83] Junghans U, Siebler M. Cerebral microembolism is blocked by tirofiban, a selective nonpeptide platelet glycoprotein IIb/IIIa receptor antagonist. Circula-tion 2003;107:2717–21.

[84] Cheung RT, Ho DS. Fatal hemorrhagic transfor-mation of acute cerebral infarction after the use of abciximab. Stroke 2000;31(10):2526–7.

[85] Deshmukh VR, Fiorella D, Albuquerque FC, et al. Intra-arterial thrombolysis for acute ischemic stroke: preliminary experience with platelet glyco-protein IIb/IIIa inhibitors as adjunctive therapy. Neurosurgery 2005;56(1):46–55.

[86] Furlan A, Higashida R, Wechsler L, et al. Intra-arterial prourokinase for acute ischemic stroke. The PROACT II study: a randomized controlled trial. Prolyse in Acute Cerebral Thromboembo-lism. JAMA 1999;282(21):2003–11.

[87] Ringer AJ, Qureshi AI, Fessler RD, et al. Angio-plasty of intracranial occlusion resistant to throm-bolysis in acute ischemic stroke. Neurosurgery 2001;48(6):1282–8.

[88] Ueda T, Sakaki S, Nochide I, et al. Angioplasty af-ter intra-arterial thrombolysis for acute occlusion of intracranial arteries. Stroke 1998;29:2568–74.

[89] Sacco RL, Foulkes MA, Mohr JP, et al. Determi-nants of early recurrence of cerebral infarction. The Stroke Data Bank. Stroke 1989;20(8):983–9.

[90] Rundek T, Elkind M, Chen X. Increased early stroke recurrence among patients with extracranial and intracranial atherosclerosis. Neurology 1998; 50:A75.

[91] Hass WK, Easton JD, Adams HP Jr, et al. A ran-domized trial comparing ticlopidine hydrochloride with aspirin for the prevention of stroke in high-risk patients. Ticlopidine Aspirin Stroke Study Group. N Engl J Med 1989;321(8):501–7.

[92] Bee JL, Bath PMW, Bousser MG, et al. Dipyrida-mole in Stroke Collaboration (DISC). Dipyrida-mole for preventing recurrent ischemic stroke and other vascular events. A meta-analysis of individ-ual patient data from randomized controlled trials. Stroke 2005;36(1):162–8.

[93] Wallace RC, Furlan AJ, Moliterno DJ, et al. Basilar artery rethrombosis: successful treatment with platelet glycoprotein IIB/IIIA receptor in-hibitor. AJNR Am J Neuroradiol 1997;18(7): 1257–60.

[94] Lempert TE, Malek AM, Halbach VV, et al. Rescue treatment of acute parent vessel thrombosis with glycoprotein IIb/IIIa inhibitor during GDC coil embolization. Stroke 1999;30(3):693–5.

[95] Tong FC, Cloft HJ, Joseph GJ, et al. Abciximab rescue in acute carotid stent thrombosis. AJNR Am J Neuroradiol 2000;21(9):1750–2.

[96] Cloft HJ, Samuels OB, Tong FC, et al. Use of abciximab for mediation of thromboembolic complications of endovascular therapy. AJNR Am J Neuroradiol 2001;22(9):1764–7.

[97] Ng PP, Phatouros CC, Khangure MS. Use of glycoprotein IIb-IIIa inhibitor for a thromboembolic complication during Guglielmi detachable coil treatment of an acutely ruptured aneurysm. AJNR Am J Neuroradiol 2001;22(9):1761–3.

[98] Duncan IC, Fourie PA. Catheter-directed intra-arterial abciximab administration for acute thrombotic occlusions during neurointerven-

tional procedures. Intervent Neuroradiol 2002; 8:159–68.

[99] Kwon OK, Lee KJ, Han MH, et al. Intraarterially administered abciximab as an adjuvant thrombolytic therapy: report of three cases. AJNR Am J Neuroradiol 2002;23(3):447–51.

[100] Alexander MJ, Duckwiler GR, Gobin YP, et al. Management of intraprocedural arterial thrombus in cerebral aneurysm embolization with abciximab: technical case report. Neurosurgery 2002;50(4): 899–901.

[101] Mounayer C, Piotin M, Baldi S, et al. Intraarterial administration of abciximab for thromboembolic events occurring during aneurysm coil placement. AJNR Am J Neuroradiol 2003;24(10):2039–43.

[102] Song JK, Niimi Y, Fernandez PM, et al. Thrombus formation during intracranial aneurysm coil placement: treatment with intra-arterial abciximab. AJNR Am J Neuroradiol 2004;25(7):1147–53.

ELSEVIER
SAUNDERS

Neurosurg Clin N Am 16 (2005) 541–545

NEUROSURGERY
CLINICS
OF NORTH AMERICA

Intensive Care Unit Management of Interventional Neuroradiology Patients

E. Sander Connolly, Jr, MD[a,b,*], Sean D. Lavine, MD[a],
Phillip M. Meyers, MD[a,c], David Palistrandt, MD[a,b],
Agusto Parra, MD[a,b], Stephan A. Mayer, MD[a,b]

[a]Department of Neurological Surgery, Columbia University Medical Center and New York-Presbyterian Hospital,
710 West 168th Street, Room 435, New York, NY 10032, USA
[b]Department of Neurology, Columbia University Medical Center and New York-Presbyterian Hospital,
710 West 168th Street, New York, NY 10032, USA
[c]Department of Radiology, Columbia University Medical Center and New York-Presbyterian Hospital,
710 West 168th Street, New York, NY 10032, USA

The management of interventional neurologic patients in the intensive care unit (ICU) is based on their underlying disease for the most part. Patients with ischemic stroke are largely managed like patients with ischemic stroke who have not undergone interventional procedures, and the same is true for those with an aneurysmal subarachnoid hemorrhage or intracerebral hemorrhage (ICH) secondary to an arteriovenous malformation, for example. Having said this, there are some special considerations that require special mention when it comes to managing patients after catheter-based procedures. Unfortunately, the data supporting these management techniques are sparse and generally of low quality. As such, much of what follows is based on less than class I data and should be viewed as no more than informed opinion.

Aneurysmal subarachnoid hemorrhage

Since the US Food and Drug Administration (FDA) approved Guglielmi detachable coils in 1995, more than 100,000 patients have had their aneurysm coiled, many of these after subarachnoid hemorrhage [1]. With the publication of the International Subarachnoid Aneurysm Trial

(ISAT) trial results in 2002, there has been an increasing shift in many centers to coil all but the most anatomically unfavorable ruptured aneurysms [2]. Despite these developments, little has been written about the specific management of these patients, leading one to believe that management of clipped and coiled patients is identical. Although the basics, such as immediate blood pressure stabilization, fluid management, use of nimodipine, ventricular drainage, and angioplasty when needed, are somewhat standardized [1], unique situations do arise with endovascularly treated patients that result in minor alterations.

Anticonvulsant drug use

Over the past few years, there is a growing realization that the risks of routine anticonvulsant drug (AED) use, especially phenytoin, probably outweigh the benefits [3]. As a result, many have advocated loading patients with AEDs only until the aneurysm is secured [4]. Others believe that comatose patients might benefit in the acute setting until a nonconvulsive status is ruled out [5]. Still others believe that patients who have undergone significant cerebral resections or have extensive cortical injury secondary to ICH or subdural hematoma should receive prophylaxis at least until the risk of vasospasm has passed [6]. Although no class I data actually exist for this patient population, we tend to use AEDs on a perioperative basis

---

* Corresponding author.
  E-mail address: escr@columbia.edu (E.S. Connolly).

in surgically treated patients but avoid their use in coiled patients.

As more data accumulate regarding the utility and risk of perioperative AEDs, differences between the management of coiled and clipped patients may disappear.

Intraventricular tissue plasminogen activator for casted ventricles

Increasingly, it has been shown that intraventricular blood is associated with a worse outcome after aneurysmal subarachnoid hemorrhage [7]. In some cases, external ventricular drain patency is threatened, leading to elevations in intracranial pressure (ICP); in other cases, massive clot burden leads to prolonged drain dependency and an increased risk of ventriculitis [8]. For these reasons, several investigators have begun to use intraventricular thrombolysis in select patients [9,10]. Although surgically clipped lesions seem to be undisturbed by these proteases, considerable debate exists with regard to lesions that have been coiled [9,11]. Although the fear seems to be more theoretic than experiential, the thought of dissolving the dome of a lesion and thereby gaining access to clot within the coil interstices continues to give many clinicians reason to pause. This fact, combined with the ability of the surgeon performing a pterional craniotomy to open the lamina terminalis with little additional effort or morbidity, has led some to advocate craniotomy over coiling in cases of casted ventricles [12].

External ventricular drainage

Although the use of external ventricular drainage in patients with subarachnoid hemorrhage is quite varied from institution to institution, there is a general feeling that patients in a coma (Hunt and Hess grades 4 and 5) benefit, as do those in better condition who have ventriculomegaly and deteriorating findings on examination [13]. Although patients in a coma are generally immediately drained to exclude increased ICP as a cause of their coma, many awake patients with ventriculomegaly, even with deteriorating examination results, are taken to the operating room before ventriculostomy and managed by other techniques, such as spinal drainage, in an effort to avoid rebleeding precipitated by changes in transmural pressure [14]. This approach still allows for placement of a ventricular drain through the craniotomy opening should the relaxation be insufficient

and has allowed several groups to report anecdotal reductions in the incidence of ventricular drainage and, by extension, ventriculitis. Still others have advocated leaving the spinal drain in after surgery, because anecdotal evidence may suggest that this leads to a diminished incidence of symptomatic vasospasm, presumably by facilitating the clearance of subarachnoid blood [15].

In contrast, endovascularly treated patients usually have drains placed before coiling if there is any ventriculomegaly whatsoever. The reason for this is twofold. First, patients who may be alert before surgery may develop increases in ICP when laid flat on the angiography table. Second, if there is any untoward event during angiography, such as might occur with aneurysm dome perforation, the delay in putting in a drain may be significant. Furthermore, if the coiling is uncomplicated but the patient experiences some major thromboembolic complication (eg, dissection, lost coil or guidewire, parent vessel thrombosis, catheter embolus), full-dose anticoagulation may be necessary. If the patient subsequently develops worsening hydrocephalus requiring drain placement, the risk of catheter-induced ICH is significant.

Antiplatelet agents

Generally speaking, patients with aneurysmal subarachnoid hemorrhage managed with craniotomy are never placed on antiplatelet agents, even if they have relatively strong indications for being on them, for fear of postoperative subdural or epidural bleeding. In addition, many patients require multiple additional invasive procedures, such as ventriculostomy, gastrostomy, tracheostomy, and central line placement. With the advent of the Neuroform stent and its use in the treatment of wide-necked aneurysms, the issue of antiplatelet therapy, particularly aspirin together with clopidogrel, has resurfaced. For the most part, it is the general feeling that when wide-necked aneurysms must be coiled in the setting of subarachnoid hemorrhage, it is better to perform the procedure with a balloon-assisted technique rather than place a stent if at all possible [16]. Residua can be dealt with later by delayed stent placement after the need for additional procedures has passed. In the case that a patient is on aspirin and clopidogrel because of stent placement, it may be feasible to reverse these drugs temporarily by fresh single-donor platelet transfusion, followed by reinstitution of the drugs after an undetermined period of watchful waiting.

Antifibrinolytic therapy

Although early trials showed this approach to reduce rebleeding at the expense of increased delayed ischemia with no improvement in overall outcome [17], recent data may suggest that ultra-early use (first 48 hours after bleeding) while the patient is being transported for definitive treatment may actually improve the outcome without increasing delayed ischemia [18]. Although those performing open craniotomy have been quick to support such an approach, especially given the evidence that immediate surgery is often less than immediate, there has been some concern among endovascular surgeons that such therapy might lead to an increase in the thromboembolic complications associated with coiling. Although there is no evidence to date that this is the case, careful assessment may require an independent assessment of the risk of these therapies in endovascularly managed patients.

Vasospasm monitoring and treatment

Although there are reports suggesting an increased, decreased, and similar incidence of vasospasm in patients managed endovascularly compared with those managed via craniotomy, there is no evidence that the medical management of coiled patients should be any different [19]. Nimodipine therapy and intravascular volume maintenance as well as the use of hypertonic saline, mannitol, and pressors for those with symptoms are essentially the same for all [1]. The early use of angioplasty and intra-arterial vasodilators in patients who fail to respond to medical maneuvers is also the same. Although part of the medical management of these patients includes optimization of blood oxygen-carrying capacity and rheology and, by extension, attention to marked anemia, most patients undergoing clipping have also undergone catheter angiography and are therefore also at risk for retroperitoneal hemorrhage. Thus, any patient with unexplained blood loss should undergo abdominal and pelvic CT scanning to rule this out. After catheter-based procedures, those patients may be at increased risk because of the use of larger guiding catheter sheaths.

Partially treated aneurysms

As long as the site of aneurysmal bleeding has been excluded from the circulation, there is little risk for acute rebleeding during the ICU stay (7–21 days). In one study in which 80% of patients were undertreated and heparin was used to guard against a thromboembolic phenomenon, there were no episodes of early rebleeding even when induced hypertension was used to treat spasm [20]. Although it is often difficult to know the exact site of the bleeding, and one can think of exceptions, patients with partially coiled aneurysms can be treated the same as those with perfectly coiled or clipped lesions. Additional unruptured aneurysms have been shown to remain unruptured in the setting of even aggressive triple-H therapy or balloon angioplasty and do not require treatment in the acute setting [21]. Occasionally, a coil may become stretched as the coiling is coming to a conclusion, leaving a tail in the efferent or afferent vessel. Usually, this requires no additional management, but if there is associated thromboembolism, aspirin (81 mg/d) is usually prescribed and platelet transfusions are used for significant invasive procedures.

Ischemic stroke

Patients with ischemic stroke are rarely transferred to the ICU unless their mental status is compromised. As a result, most of the ischemic strokes that are managed are caused by large-vessel thromboembolism and are being treated as part of acute stroke protocols. These protocols include the FDA-approved use of intravenous tissue plasminogen activator (rt-PA) for those presenting within 3 hours as well as the non–FDA-approved use of intra-arterial rt-PA or urokinase within 6 hours [22–24]. For those who receive intravenous rt-PA but do not recanalize, "bridging protocols" have been developed to allow for the subsequent use of intra-arterial "lytics" within 6 hours. For those who still do not recanalize or for those presenting with large areas of perfusion-diffusion "mismatch" on perfusion-weighted imaging or diffusion-weighted imaging MRI, the FDA has approved the use of a mechanical endovascular corkscrew [25,26]. This has been used out to 8 hours in the anterior circulation with varied success and out to 12 to 18 hours in the posterior circulation. In terms of ICU management, patients are initially kept hypertensive until recanalization is achieved and their pressure is then lowered. Ideally, patients are managed with a combination of anticoagulation and antiplatelet therapy (aspirin and clopidogrel) unless the infarct area is greater than 30 to 40 mL. With these larger infarcts, especially when reperfusion is successful, we have generally gone with antiplatelet therapy alone for fear of inducing hemorrhagic conversion of the infarcted tissue.

Patients who ultimately develop large hemispheric strokes have been treated with surgical decompression as well as aggressive medical therapy depending on family desires [27]. The early data from the small but randomized, prospective, multicenter trial for hemicraniectomy seem to suggest a survival advantage but no improvement in function [28]. Moreover, hemicraniectomy is not benign and has been associated with a whole host of side effects that are difficult to manage, such as hydrocephalus, wound breakdown, meningitis, and even delayed epidural bleeding. Patient selection for this procedure is therefore key [29]. Meta-analysis suggests that younger patients, especially those with massive swelling despite incomplete middle cerebral artery territory infarction, specifically that involving the nondominant hemisphere, may be best served [30]. For others, we have used a combination of mild (34.5 °C–35.5 °C) prolonged (7–10 days) hypothermia together with hypertonic saline (2% and 3%), followed by gradual withdrawal of both [31]. Dramatic anecdotal successes exist, but there are an equally large number of patients who have not responded.

General

For patients with hemorrhage as well as ischemic stroke, significant efforts are made to maintain normal magnesium and glucose levels, with frequent testing and intravenous drips when necessary. These efforts are based on strong data for magnesium in animal models as well as in human beings with eclampsia, neonatal birth injury, and subarachnoid hemorrhage [32]. The data for normoglycemia are class I but were acquired in patients with a whole host of injuries (not just those to the nervous system) [33]. In addition, although hypothermia is used experimentally in the ICU, normothermia and the avoidance of fever are generally considered a "good idea" for all neurologically injured patients [34]. This comes from the fact that hyperthermia is closely associated in multivariate models with a poor outcome after ischemia and hemorrhagic stroke [34]. As a result, patients are managed with a variety of surface-cooling devices (eg, blankets, pads) until such time that failure necessitates intravascular cooling with a variety of FDA-approved and non–FDA-approved devices. Although studies have not randomized patients to

device-maintained normothermia or placebo, such studies are currently being organized and should provide ample support for these efforts going forward [34,35].

Summary

The ICU management of patients undergoing endovascular procedures is complex and varied. It depends not only on the underlying disease process but on the exact nature of the procedure performed, the procedure's success, and whether or not there were any procedural complications, however minor. As a result, there are few class I data to support much of what is done. In fact, most management techniques are drawn from other settings and anecdotal experience. We have highlighted just a few of the issues that arise.

As an increasing number of endovascularly treated patients find their way into ICUs, it should be increasingly important to examine whether the treatments used are ideal and, if not, how they can be improved on. This is likely to require multicenter collaboration as well as a change in the way society views the neurologically injured patient. Currently, many states prohibit the enrollment of comatose patients into randomized clinical trials because they do not recognize next of kin assent as sufficient. We can only hope that as the debate rages over quality in health care, comatose patients are also allowed to participate in the fruits of evidenced-based approaches.

References

[1] Wijdicks EF, Kallmes DF, Manno EM, et al. Subarachnoid hemorrhage: neurointensive care and aneurysm repair. Mayo Clin Proc 2005;80:550–9.
[2] Molyneux A, Kerr R, Stratton I, et al. International Subarachnoid Aneurysm Trial (ISAT) of neurosurgical clipping versus endovascular coiling in 2143 patients with ruptured intracranial aneurysms: a randomised trial. Lancet 2002;360:1267–74.
[3] Naidech AM, Kreiter KT, Janjua N, et al. Phenytoin exposure is associated with functional and cognitive disability after subarachnoid hemorrhage. Stroke 2005;36:583–7.
[4] Baker CJ, Prestigiacomo CJ, Solomon RA. Short-term perioperative anticonvulsant prophylaxis for the surgical treatment of low-risk patients with intracranial aneurysms. Neurosurgery 1995;37:863–70.
[5] Claassen J, Peery S, Kreiter KT, et al. Predictors and clinical impact of epilepsy after subarachnoid hemorrhage. Neurology 2003;60:208–14.
[6] Claassen J, Mayer SA, Kowalski RG, et al. Detection of electrographic seizures with continuous

EEG monitoring in critically ill patients. Neurology 2004;62:1743–8.

[7] Claassen J, Bernardini GL, Kreiter K, et al. Effect of cisternal and ventricular blood on risk of delayed cerebral ischemia after subarachnoid hemorrhage: the Fisher scale revisited. Stroke 2001;32: 2012–20.

[8] Lozier AP, Sciacca RR, Romagnoli MF, et al. Ventriculostomy-related infections: a critical review of the literature. Neurosurgery 2002;51:170–81.

[9] Findlay JM, Jacka MJ. Cohort study of intraventricular thrombolysis with recombinant tissue plasminogen activator for aneurysmal intraventricular hemorrhage. Neurosurgery 2004;55:532–7.

[10] Naff NJ, Hanley DF, Keyl PM, et al. Intraventricular thrombolysis speeds blood clot resolution: results of a pilot, prospective, randomized, double-blind, controlled trial. Neurosurgery 2004;54:577–83.

[11] Azmi-Ghadimi H, Heary RF, Farkas JE, et al. Use of intraventricular tissue plasminogen activator and Guglielmi detachable coiling for the acute treatment of casted ventricles from cerebral aneurysm hemorrhage: two technical case reports. Neurosurgery 2002;50:421–4.

[12] Findlay JM, Weir BK, Kassell NF, et al. Intracisternal recombinant tissue plasminogen activator after aneurysmal subarachnoid hemorrhage. J Neurosurg 1991;75:181–8.

[13] Le Roux PD, Elliott JP, Newell DW, et al. Predicting outcome in poor-grade patients with subarachnoid hemorrhage: a retrospective review of 159 aggressively managed cases. J Neurosurg 1996;85: 39–49.

[14] Connolly ES Jr, Kader AA, Frazzini VI, et al. The safety of intraoperative lumbar subarachnoid drainage for acutely ruptured intracranial aneurysm: technical note. Surg Neurol 1997;48:338–42.

[15] Klimo P Jr, Kestle JR, MacDonald JD, et al. Marked reduction of cerebral vasospasm with lumbar drainage of cerebrospinal fluid after subarachnoid hemorrhage. J Neurosurg 2004;100:215–24.

[16] Han PP, Albuquerque FC, Ponce FA, et al. Percutaneous intracranial stent placement for aneurysms. J Neurosurg 2003;99:23–30.

[17] Kassell NF, Torner JC, Adams HP Jr. Antifibrinolytic therapy in the acute period following aneurysmal subarachnoid hemorrhage. Preliminary observations from the Cooperative Aneurysm Study. J Neurosurg 1984;61:225–30.

[18] Hillman J, Fridriksson S, Nilsson O, et al. Immediate administration of tranexamic acid and reduced incidence of early rebleeding after aneurysmal subarachnoid hemorrhage: a prospective randomized study. J Neurosurg 2002;97:771–8.

[19] Hohlrieder M, Spiegel M, Hinterhoelzl J, et al. Cerebral vasospasm and ischaemic infarction in clipped and coiled intracranial aneurysm patients. Eur J Neurol 2002;9:389–99.

[20] Bernardini GL, Mayer SA, Kossoff SB, et al. Anticoagulation and induced hypertension after endovascular treatment for ruptured intracranial aneurysms. Crit Care Med 2001;29:641–4.

[21] Swift DM, Solomon RA. Unruptured aneurysms and postoperative volume expansion. J Neurosurg 1992;77:908–10.

[22] National Institute of Neurological Disorders and Stroke rt-PA Stroke Study Group. Tissue plasminogen activator for acute ischemic stroke. N Engl J Med 1995;333:1581–7.

[23] del Zoppo GJ, Higashida RT, Furlan AJ, et al. PROACT: a phase II randomized trial of recombinant pro-urokinase by direct arterial delivery in acute middle cerebral artery stroke. PROACT Investigators. Prolyse in Acute Cerebral Thromboembolism. Stroke 1998;29:4–11.

[24] Wardlaw JM. Overview of Cochrane thrombolysis meta-analysis. Neurology 2001;57(Suppl):S69–76.

[25] Becker KJ, Brott TG. Approval of the MERCI clot retriever: a critical view. Stroke 2005;36:400–3.

[26] Gobin YP, Starkman S, Duckwiler GR, et al. MERCI 1: a phase 1 study of mechanical embolus removal in cerebral ischemia. Stroke 2004;35:2848–54.

[27] Mayer SA, Kossoff SB. Withdrawal of life support in the neurological intensive care unit. Neurology 1999;52:1602–9.

[28] Fandino J, Keller E, Barth A, et al. Decompressive craniotomy after middle cerebral artery infarction. Retrospective analysis of patients treated in three centres in Switzerland. Swiss Med Wkly 2004;134: 423–9.

[29] Curry WT Jr, Sethi MK, Ogilvy CS, et al. Factors associated with outcome after hemicraniectomy for large middle cerebral artery territory infarction. Neurosurgery 2005;56:681–92.

[30] Gupta R, Connolly ES, Mayer S, et al. Hemicraniectomy for massive middle cerebral artery territory infarction: a systematic review. Stroke 2004; 35:539–43.

[31] Georgiadis D, Schwarz S, Aschoff A, et al. Hemicraniectomy and moderate hypothermia in patients with severe ischemic stroke. Stroke 2000;33: 1584–8.

[32] van den Bergh WM. Magnesium sulfate in aneurysmal subarachnoid hemorrhage. A randomized controlled trial. Stroke 2005.

[33] van den Berghe G, Wouters P, Weekers F, et al. Intensive insulin therapy in the critically ill patients. N Engl J Med 2001;345:1359–67.

[34] Mayer SA, Kowalski RG, Presciutti M, et al. Clinical trial of a novel surface cooling system for fever control in neurocritical care patients. Crit Care Med 2004;32:2508–15.

[35] Mayer S, Commichau C, Scarmeas N, et al. Clinical trial of an air-circulating cooling blanket for fever control in critically ill neurologic patients. Neurology 2001;56:292–8.

NEUROSURGERY
CLINICS
OF NORTH AMERICA

Neurosurg Clin N Am 16 (2005) 547–560

Interventional Neuroradiology Adjuncts and Alternatives in Patients with Head and Neck Vascular Lesions

Michele H. Johnson, MD[a],*, Veronica L. Chiang, MD[b],
Douglas A. Ross, MD[c]

[a]Interventional Neuroradiology, Department of Diagnostic Radiology, Yale University School of Medicine,
333 Cedar Street, PO Box 8042, New Haven, CT 06520–8042, USA
[b]Department of Neurosurgery, Yale University School of Medicine, 333 Cedar Street,
PO Box 8082, New Haven, CT 06520, USA
[c]Section of Otolaryngology, Department of Surgery, Yale University School of Medicine,
333 Cedar Street, PO Box 8041, New Haven, CT 06520, USA

Endovascular techniques can be applied to a variety of benign and malignant extracranial lesions of the head, neck, and skull base. We discuss the role of endovascular techniques in the management of benign and malignant head and neck neoplasms, acute and delayed presentations of vascular traumatic injury, and acute management of head and neck bleeding. We discuss endovascular options and management strategies for treatment of extracranial lesions of the head, neck, and skull base.

Neoplastic disease

Benign and malignant tumors may compromise head and neck vascular supply or derive significant neovascularity from the extracranial vasculature. In most cases, a CT scan with or without the addition of CT angiography (CTA) or MRI with MR angiography (MRA) can demonstrate the relation of the mass to the vasculature, provide a differential diagnosis, and provide an opportunity for image-guided biopsy. Catheter angiography is reserved for those cases in which significant neovascularity is expected or where the potential for major vessel compromise is present, requiring a temporary balloon occlusion tolerance test (BTO) or major vessel sacrifice before en bloc resection [1–5].

Benign neoplasms

Benign tumors of the head, neck, and skull base may compress, displace, or encase the carotid or vertebral arteries, making complete resection difficult. Successful preoperative BTO of the carotid or vertebral artery before surgery may provide the surgeon with increased assurance in surgical planning and patient counseling. Schwannoma and neurofibroma of the neck or skull base, paraganglioma (carotid body tumor, glomus vagale, or glomus jugulare), and esthesioneuroblastoma or meningioma with a significant extracranial component as well as tumors with significant cavernous sinus extension may benefit from preoperative BTO [6,7].

Preoperative BTO of the vertebral artery may be followed by preoperative vertebral artery sacrifice before resection of aggressive benign spine tumors, such as osteoblastoma or an aneurysmal bone cyst (Fig. 1) [8].

Temporary balloon occlusion tolerance test

BTO is composed of an angiographic anatomic and clinical neurologic assessment of a patient's

---

* Corresponding author.
E-mail address: michele.h.johnson@yale.edu
(M.H. Johnson).

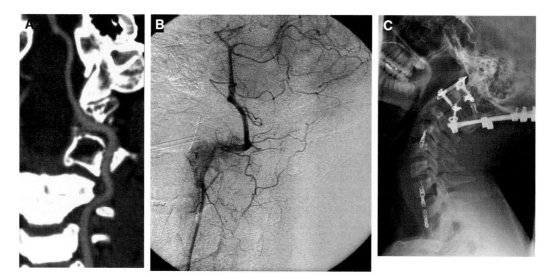

Fig. 1. (*A–C*) CTA shows patent vertebral artery encased by osseous C_2 tumor (T). Vertebral angiogram reveals a hypervascular mass. Preoperative vertebral artery sacrifice using platinum microcoils was performed in this adolescent with C1 osteoblastoma.

ability to tolerate temporary occlusion of a major vessel [6,7,9,10]. The components include a diagnostic arteriogram to assess anatomic collaterals, administration of heparin before inflation of a contrast-containing nondetachable balloon with occlusion of the major vessel, and clinical neurologic testing while the balloon is inflated for approximately 30 minutes. If the patient tolerates the normotensive temporary occlusion, hypotension may be pharmacologically induced with reduction of the mean arterial pressure (MAP) to two thirds of the baseline blood pressure and extending the temporary occlusion for an additional 15 minutes. This hypotensive challenge is analogous to a stress or exercise state and may unmask subtle hypoperfusion. For BTO of the anterior circulation, the predictive value can be improved by the injection of the radionuclide Tc99m hexamethylpropyleneamine-oxime (HM-PAO; exametazime) before brain single photon emission CT (SPECT) imaging [9]. Tc99m HM-PAO is a single-pass blood flow agent that provides a snapshot of cerebral blood flow at the time of injection. Cerebral SPECT imaging can take place up to 6 hours after injection and reflects the cerebral blood flow at the time of hypotension and BTO of the major vessel (Fig. 2). After injection of Tc99m HM-PAO, the balloon is deflated, antihypertensive medication is discontinued, and blood flow is restored to the cerebral circulation. SPECT imaging is of lesser value

for assessment of the posterior fossa after vertebral artery temporary occlusion and is rarely performed.

The predictive value of tolerance BTO of the internal carotid artery with a combination of angiographic demonstration of anatomic collaterals, normotensive and hypotensive clinical tolerance of test occlusion, and satisfactory perfusion on brain SPECT is approximately 85% that the patient can tolerate permanent occlusion without infarction [10–12]. Risks of the test occlusion include stroke and local blood vessel injury in addition to the overall risks of cerebral angiography.

Preoperative embolization is commonly used for juvenile nasal angiofibroma, esthesioneuroblastoma, meningioma, schwannoma, neurofibroma, and paraganglioma. Preoperative particulate embolization using polyvinyl alcohol (PVA) foam particles measuring 250 to 350 μm in size 1 to 2 days before surgical excision increases safety by decreasing blood loss at the time of surgery and thus facilitates a safer and more complete resection. The embolization can be performed in the same angiographic day following BTO and SPECT (Fig. 3) [3,4].

Extracranial transarterial tumor embolization adds a small risk to the performance of cerebral angiography. The principal risks include blood vessel injury and stroke. With some tumors of the skull base, there is a risk of opening potential collaterals between the extracranial and intracranial

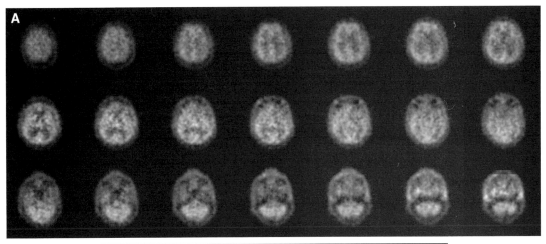

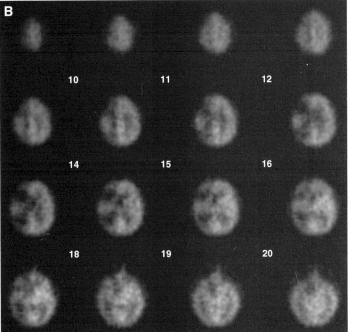

Fig. 2. Temporary carotid balloon occlusion test (BTO) is performed with a contrast-filled non-detachable balloon catheter. Tc99m HM-PAO is injected during temporary occlusion. (A) SPECT following carotid BTO demonstrates no differential cerebral hemisphere hypoperfusion. (B) SPECT demonstrates marked hypoperfusion in a patient with massive carotid bleeding following urgent endovascular occlusion.

circulations, such as the inferolateral trunk and the vidian artery (internal maxillary artery to internal carotid artery) or middle meningeal artery to ophthalmic artery during the embolization procedure resulting in cerebral emboli. Similarly, extracranial-to-intracranial anastomoses occur between the vertebral artery and the ascending pharyngeal and occipital arteries [2,5]. Extracranial tumoral embolization is well tolerated by patients, although they may experience some increase in pain in the region of a large tumor mass resulting from tumoral ischemia and edema after embolization.

Malignant neoplasms

Malignant neoplasms of head and neck origin predominantly include tumors of squamous cell

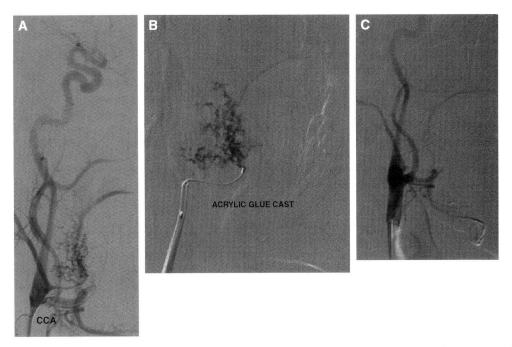

Fig. 3. (A–C) Preoperative embolization of a large, hypervascular, parapharyngeal space schwannoma using a combination of PVA particles and acrylic.

origin involving the paranasal sinuses, oral-digestive tract, or larynx. Adenocarcinomas and mucoepidermoid carcinomas arising from minor salivary glands as well as other more unusual tumors may arise in this region. Many of these lesions extend to involve the skull base and create symptoms in the central nervous system. Most of these malignancies are relatively hypovascular, with the exception of malignant paraganglioma; thus, most do not require preoperative embolization. In large tumors adjacent to the carotid artery, en bloc resection may require sacrifice of the carotid artery [3]. BTO followed by endovascular carotid sacrifice 3 to 6 weeks before en bloc resection is associated with a lower stroke risk than is surgical carotid sacrifice at the time of en bloc resection [6]. The interval of a few weeks allows re-equilibration of the cerebral blood flow before the stress of major surgical resection. After endovascular carotid sacrifice, these patients are managed in the neurointensive care unit with heparin therapy and control of fluid dynamics to decrease stroke risk during the equilibration period. There is limited experience with intra-arterial administration of chemotherapeutic agents into locally recurrent or locally advanced and unresectable tumors [13–17]. Despite significant local toxicity, early results suggest tumor regression that may permit salvage surgery. These techniques have not yet become the standard of care for advanced head and neck cancers.

Carotid blow-out syndrome

Many of these patients receive intraoperative brachytherapy as part of their tumor management. The combination of malignant disease recurrence, surgery, and radiation therapy may result in vascular injury with tumoral encasement, vessel wall ulceration, or pseudoaneurysm formation. Radiation injury to the carotid and or vertebral arteries in the neck may result in symptomatic stenosis and present with transient ischemic attack (TIA) or stroke, even without residual tumor (Fig. 4). Patients more commonly present with acute oral, nasal, or paratracheal bleeding weeks to months after the initial presentation and surgery. The exact site of injury relates to the location of the tumor in relation to the major vessels, the degree of intrinsic tumoral vascularity, the presence of tumoral or mucosal ulcerations, and the types of prior treatment. Localization of surgical clips or brachytherapy seeds is a good indication of the site of potential

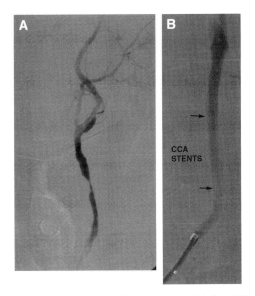

Fig. 4. (*A*) After successful treatment of left middle cerebral stroke with intravenous tissue plasminogen activator, angiography revealed left common carotid stenosis 12 years after radiation therapy for laryngeal carcinoma. (*B*) Two overlapping stents were placed.

vascular injury leading to hemorrhage. When the oral, nasal, or paratracheal bleeding is mild to moderate, it may result from erosion through the wall of a small vessel and can usually be treated with vessel-specific embolization with particles or acrylic designed to maintain patency of the major vessels.

The term *carotid blow-out* (CBO) specifically refers to catastrophic rupture of the common, internal, or external carotid artery or their branches with life-threatening hemorrhage [18–23]. Rapid initiation of resuscitation securing airway followed by oral or nasal packing and angiography with endovascular occlusive techniques may be lifesaving (Fig. 5). For carotid rupture, the standard of care is sacrifice of the carotid artery above and below the point of rupture. It is important to include areas of intimal irregularity as demonstrated on angiography or, alternatively, to span the region of vessel encasement as visualized on cross-sectional imaging. Carotid occlusion by detachable balloons has been the mainstay of therapy, although these are currently unavailable in the United States. Alternatively, platinum microcoils, usually a combination of detachable and complex helical coils, can be

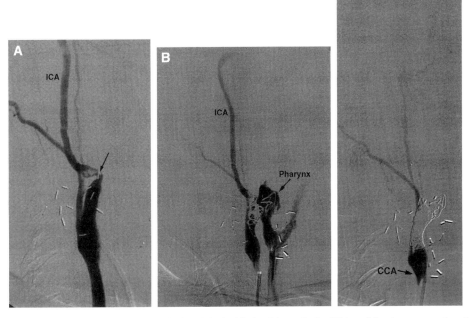

Fig. 5. (*A–C*) CBO with permanent coil occlusion. Marked intimal irregularity ICA and frank extravasation from the internal cartoid into the pharynx in a patient with recurrent squamous cell carcinoma of the hypopharynx.

used for effective carotid occlusion. A combination of platinum and fibered platinum coils can be used to promote effective and rapid occlusion. Even when frank rupture is not demonstrated angiographically, the treatment of a pseudoaneurysm and ulceration in the common or internal carotid artery usually requires carotid sacrifice. Resuscitation and packing usually allow enough time for rapid angiographic assessment of the circle of Willis before endovascular occlusion. When lifesaving carotid sacrifice must be performed without preocclusion testing, HM-PAO SPECT may be performed after the occlusion to assist in planning for aggressive hypertensive and hypervolemic management [6,7,10].

We have had limited experience with good success at our institution in treating patients without adequate circle of Willis collaterals with covered stents to cover the area of vascular injury and to preserve cerebral blood flow. This technique is experimental, and there are significant limitations in terms of the size and length of available stents (generally approved for biliary or tracheobronchial use). Increased availability of stents in smaller (<5 mm) diameters and longer (>5 cm) lengths may allow more widespread application of this cerebral perfusion–saving technology to this group of critically ill patients (Fig. 6) [18,20,21].

Traumatic vascular injuries

Vascular injury from blunt or penetrating trauma may present acutely with expanding hematoma or oral or nasal bleeding or may present in a delayed fashion, such as in the development of a pseudoaneurysm or carotid cavernous fistula [24–28]. A CT scan, with or without adjunctive CTA, is useful for defining the location of fracture fragments or the path of a projectile and may demonstrate the injury before endovascular or surgical treatment. Angiography may demonstrate vessel laceration, vasospasm, dissection, occlusion, or pseudoaneurysm formation, with or without distal embolization. Oral or nasal bleeding secondary to facial fractures may initially be treated by packing in the emergency room, followed by angiographic evaluation of the common, internal, and external carotid arteries and their branches. Transarterial embolization is performed similar to that described for idiopathic epistaxis. Temporary agents, such as Gelfoam pledgets (Pharmacia & Upjohn, Kalamazoo, Michigan) or larger PVA foam particles (250–350 μm or 300–500 μm), are useful to provide immediate hemostasis and to allow healing without compromising facial arterial supply

Vertebral artery injury most commonly results from cervical spine fractures caused by blunt or

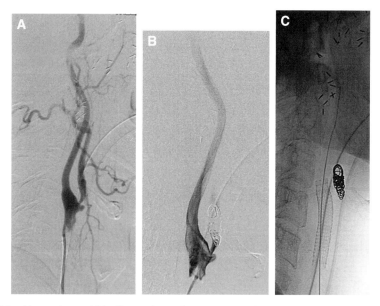

Fig. 6. (A–C) CBO with massive oral bleeding and pseudoaneurysm at the carotid bulb. Fibered coils were placed to exclude the proximal external carotid artery before covered stent placement in the common and internal cartoid artery with cessation of bleeding.

penetrating injury with resultant dissection, occlusion, pseudoaneurysm, or fistula formation. The vertebral artery is especially vulnerable to injury at the anatomic points of fixation, such as the entrance into the foramen transversarium at C5 to C6, the junction of C1 and C2, and above C1, where the vertebral artery pierces the dura. CTA at the time of the initial CT scan may demonstrate loss of integrity of the transverse foramen and demonstrate the concomitant vascular injury. Persistent antegrade flow in dissected or partially occluded vertebral arteries may lead to distal embolization and stroke. Heparin with or without antiplatelet therapy has become the mainstay of treatment for such patients, although vertebral artery sacrifice remains a viable treatment strategy to prevent distal embolization in patients with adequate posterior circulation collateral flow (carotid arteries and contralateral vertebral artery). Stent technology is not an important form of treatment for vertebral artery injury. This is largely related to the small size of the vertebral artery and the difficulty in maintaining stent patency in small vessels.

A vertebral-jugular fistula most commonly results from penetrating trauma and may be associated with local cervical hematoma and hemodynamic instability. Transarterial embolization, usually resulting in sacrifice of the ipsilateral vertebral artery, may be curative and is well tolerated if adequate collateral circulation is present. Rarely, a venous endovascular approach or direct surgical repair is necessary for control.

Carotid artery injury may result from direct injury to the carotid and neck or may be the result of a skull base fracture with arterial dissection [24–29]. As with the vertebral artery, fixation points, such as the skull base, where the carotid pierces the dura, and within the cavernous sinus, render the carotid at the skull base more vulnerable to injury. Mandibular fractures are commonly associated with common or proximal internal carotid artery injury. Direct trauma to the common carotid artery may result in dissection or pseudoaneurysm formation with or without distal embolization (Fig. 7). Similarly, dissection leading to occlusion or pseudoaneurysm formation may occur with injuries of the internal carotid artery. A pseudoaneurysm of the internal carotid artery may be treated expectantly with antiplatelet agents, with or without heparin as for vertebral injuries. A pseudoaneurysm of the common carotid artery is generally treated by surgical repair or by endovascular treatment with bare or covered stents to

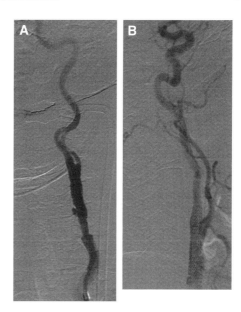

Fig. 7. (*A*) Common and internal carotid dissection secondary to seatbelt injury during a motor vehicle accident. (*B*) The patient was treated with two overlapping stents and antiplatelet therapy.

maintain distal intracranial supply [30–35]. Surgical repair of pseudoaneurysms may be curative, but access may be difficult when the aneurysm is located near the skull base or behind the mandible. Endovascular treatment, particularly with covered stent technology, can be useful in this setting. The use of antiplatelet therapy at the time of stent placement is critical to diminish platelet adhesion in the setting of vascular injury. A pseudoaneurysm of the internal carotid artery may also present in a delayed fashion as a localized mass, with local pain or Horner's syndrome. We have found CTA useful for following patients with a pseudoaneurysm on antiplatelet therapy before intervention (Fig. 8).

Traumatic carotid cavernous fistula

Delayed development of a traumatic carotid cavernous fistula is a known complication of closed-head injury. Unlike patients with vertebral-jugular fistulas, these patients do not present with hematoma or hemodynamic instability; instead, they present with proptosis or chemosis, with or without diplopia. Patients may develop increased intraocular pressure leading to visual impairment. Emergency treatment is rarely

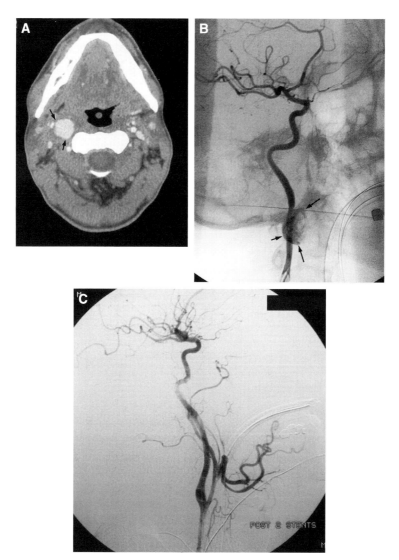

Fig. 8. (*A–C*) Intimal dissection and pseudoaneurysm (*arrows*) 1 month after motor vehicle accident seen on CT for neck mass. Angiography was followed by overlapping stent placement with exclusion of the pseudoaneurysm.

indicated, except in the setting of impending visual loss. Endovascular treatment may include closure of the fistula via an arterial approach (detachable balloons or platinum microcoils) or, alternatively, closure of the fistula via a venous approach (petrosal sinus or superior ophthalmic vein approach with platinum microcoils). The endovascular approach is dictated by the anatomy of the fistulous communication. In some cases, the severity of the carotid injury may lead to parent artery occlusion at the time of fistula treatment (Fig. 9) [36–38].

Intraoperative and perioperative vascular compromise

Intraoperative and perioperative vascular compromise may occur either during direct vascular surgery, such as an endarterectomy, or may occur in any setting in which tumor surrounds major vascular structures, that often alters the normal anatomic position and relations to adjacent structures [37–42]. The sphenoid sinus has a close relation to the internal carotid artery at its lateral and superior walls. The bone can be particularly

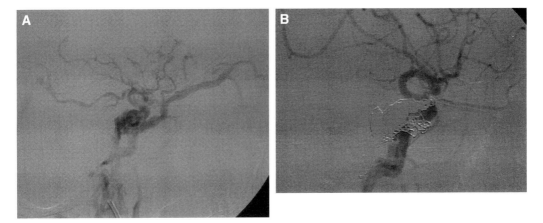

Fig. 9. (*A,B*) Carotid cavernous fistula developing after a fall was treated transvenously with coils via the petrosal sinus.

thin overlying the carotid and may be distorted in the presence of tumor or inflammatory disease. Trans-sphenoidal surgery for intrinsic sphenoid pathologic findings or for pituitary tumor removal may result in injury to the adjacent internal carotid artery, leading to hemorrhage, pseudoaneurysm, or occlusion (Figs. 10 and 11) [40]. Infection or tumor invasion involving the internal carotid at the skull base may result in similar pathologic findings (Fig. 12). Intraoperative measures to control bleeding locally are instituted in addition to sphenoid sinus packing before angiographic assessment. Endovascular repair may require carotid artery sacrifice after assessment of the remaining cerebral vasculature for adequacy

of the circle of Willis. In most cases, the incomplete wall of the pseudoaneurysm in the face of injury is too fragile for coil embolization to prevent the possibility of rupture. Currently available covered stents may not be small enough or flexible enough to negotiate the curves of the petrous and cavernous internal carotid segments routinely [38]. Parent vessel occlusion remains the mainstay of treatment for most postsurgical vascular injuries.

After placement of screws and plates for facial fracture fixation or, occasionally, after tracheostomy insertion, oral or peritracheal bleeding may occur. In the acute postoperative period (5–10 days after surgery), vascular injury with laceration

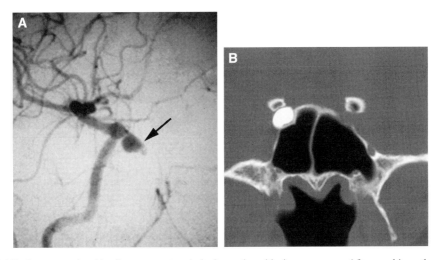

Fig. 10. (*A,B*) Intraoperative bleeding encountered during sphenoid sinus surgery. After packing, the angiogram revealed a pseudoaneurysm (*arrow*) treated with carotid occlusion. CT demonstrates the occlusive coil pack occlusion balloon position relative to the sphenoid sinus.

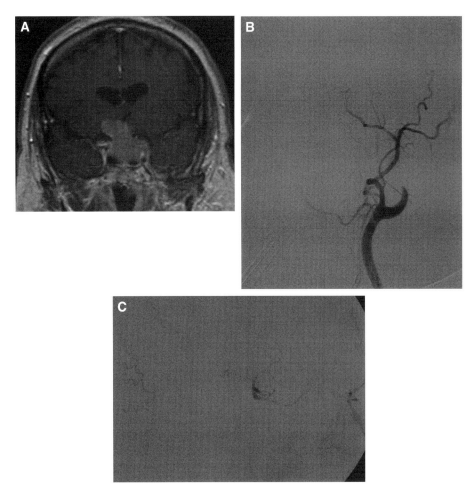

Fig. 11. (*A*) Intraoperative bleeding encountered during transphenoidal hypophysectomy for a large pituitary tumor seen on MRI. After packing, angiography revealed carotid occlusion (*B*) and poor circle of Willis collaterals on the intracranial view (*C*).

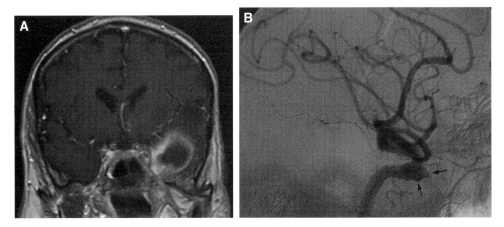

Fig. 12. (*A*) Controlled intraoperative bleeding encountered during removal of a medial temporal lobe abscess, seen on MRI, associated with mucoepidermoid carcinoma. Angiography showed minor intimal irregularity (not shown). (*B*) Massive oral bleeding occurred 5 months later; revealed a pseudoaneurysm (*arrows*) which was treated by carotid occlusion.

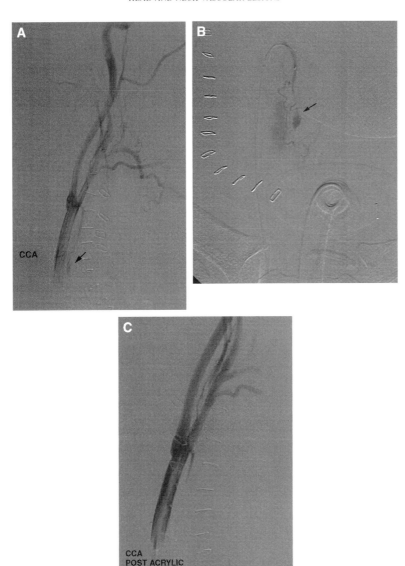

Fig. 13. Peritracheal bleeding occurred 9 days after bilateral radical neck surgery and tracheostomy. Common carotid angiography (*A*) faintly demonstrates a superior thyroidal pseudoaneurysm better seen on microcatheterization (*B*). (*C*) It was embolized with acrylic.

and a secondary pseudoaneurysm is the most commonly identified angiographic abnormality. Embolization of the lesion using particulate embolic material (PVA foam particles, Gelfoam, or coils) or, in the setting of an end artery, acrylic glue is usually efficacious for bleeding control (Fig. 13).

TIAs or hemiparesis after carotid endarterectomy may result from carotid occlusion, often requiring reoperation. Emergent angiography or, more currently, CTA may be performed to establish the cause of the symptomatology and the nature of the vascular compromise before surgical re-exploration. Stent technology might also be applied in this postsurgical setting.

Epistaxis and other endovascular interventions in the head and neck

When no traumatic, neoplastic, or intrinsic vascular cause for epistaxis is identified, it is referred to as idiopathic. Epistaxis may require

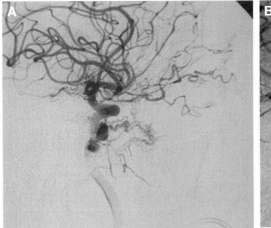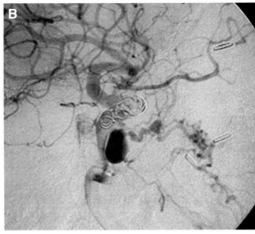

Fig. 14. (*A,B*) CBO with massive bleeding in an 80-year-old patient with HHT and multiple prior external cartoid branch ligations (clips). He had had multiple prior embolizations and developed this internal carotid pseudoaneurysm and extensive nasal collaterals, seen most clearly after partial carotid occlusion. Internal carotid coil occlusion resulted in cessation of bleeding.

endovascular treatment when posterior packs fail to control the bleeding [3,4,43]. Transarterial embolization consists of distal particulate embolization (PVA foam particles measuring 250–355 μm) in the distal internal maxillary artery and distal facial artery on the ipsilateral side and embolization of the distal internal maxillary or facial artery on the contralateral side, reserving a single branch to maintain adequate collateral blood supply to the nasal tissues. Transarterial embolization is well tolerated and highly effective in the idiopathic epistaxis patient population, with a low complication rate (2%).

Hereditary hemorrhagic telangiectasia (HHT) is an autosomal dominant vascular dysplasia with telangiectasia of the nasal and gastrointestinal mucosa, skin, and respiratory tract as well as arteriovenous malformations of the lung, liver, and brain [44]. Epistaxis may be difficult to control endovascularly (Fig. 14). Septal dermoplasty has been found to be more effective and durable in the management of transfusion-dependent epistaxis [45].

Summary

Vascular lesions of the head and neck include a variety of neoplastic and traumatic lesions that may cause local neurologic symptoms or may compromise the carotid or vertebral arteries, leading to ischemic deficits. Management of lesions involving vascular structures at the skull

base may require BTO or endovascular transarterial embolization as part of the preoperative evaluation. Endovascular techniques can be used as a salvage measure for severe head and neck bleeding and can assist with the management of vascular injury occurring in the operative or perioperative setting. Familiarity with the role of endovascular techniques in this group of patients may favorably influence patient management and outcome.

References

[1] Johnson MH. Head and neck vascular anatomy. Neuroimaging Clin N Am 1998;8:119–41.

[2] Berenstein A, Lasjaunias P, ter Brugge K. Surgical neuroangiography: functional anatomy of craniofacial arteries. New York: Springer-Verlag; 1987/2004.

[3] Low YM, Goh YH. Intra-arterial embolization in otolaryngology—a four-year review. Singapore Med J 2003;44(6):323–4.

[4] Johnson MH. Vascular lesions of the paranasal sinuses and nasal cavity. Semin Ultrasound CT MR 1999;20:426–44.

[5] Mishkin MM, Schreiber MN. Collateral circulation. In: Newton TH, Potts DG, editors. Angiography. Radiology of the skull and brain, vol. 2, book 4. St. Louis, MO: Mosby-Year Book; 1977. p. 2344–74.

[6] Lee S, Huddle D, Awad IA. Indications and management strategies in therapeutic carotid occlusion. Neurosurgery Quarterly 2000;10:211–23.

[7] Dare AO, Gibbons KJ, Gillihan MD, et al. Hypotensive endovascular test occlusion of the carotid ar-

tery in head and neck cancer. Neurosurg Focus 2003;
14(3):1–4.

[8] Bilsky MH, Boakye M, Collignon F, et al. Operative management of metastatic and malignant primary subaxial cervical tumors. J Neurosurg Spine 2005; 2(3):256–64.

[9] Palestro CJ, Sen C, Muzinic M, et al. Assessing collateral cerebral perfusion with technetium-99m-HMPAO SPECT during temporary internal carotid artery occlusion. J Nucl Med 1994;35(9):1556–7.

[10] Dare AO, Chaloupka JC, Putman CM, et al. Failure of the hypotensive provocative test during temporary balloon test occlusion of the internal carotid artery to predict delayed hemodynamic ischemia after therapeutic carotid occlusion. Surg Neurol 1998; 50(2):147–55.

[11] Charbel FT, Zhao M, Amin-Hanjani S, et al. A patient-specific computer model to predict outcomes of the balloon occlusion test. J Neurosurg 2004;101(6): 977–88.

[12] McIvor NP, Willinsky RA, TerBrugge KG, et al. Validity of test occlusion studies prior to internal carotid artery sacrifice. Head Neck 1994;15:11–6.

[13] Balm AJM, Rasch CRN, Schornagel JH, et al. High-dose superselective intra-arterial cisplatin and concomitant radiation (radplat) for advanced head and neck cancer. Head Neck 2004;26(6): 485–93.

[14] Kovacs AF. Intra-arterial induction high-dose chemotherapy with cisplatin for oral and oropharyngeal cancer: long-term results. Br J Cancer 2004;90(7): 1323–8.

[15] Kerber CW, Wong WH, Howell SB, et al. An organ-preserving selective arterial chemotherapy strategy for head and neck cancer. AJNR Am J Neuroradiol 1998;19:935–41.

[16] Robbins KT, Kumar P, Harris J, et al. Supradose intra-arterial cisplatin and concurrent radiation therapy for the treatment of stage IV head and neck squamous cell carcinoma is feasible and efficacious in a multi-institutional setting: results of Radiation Therapy Oncology Group Trial 9615. J Clin Oncol 2005;23(7):1447–54.

[17] Robbins KT. Is high-dose intensity intraarterial cisplatin chemoradiotherapy for head and neck carcinoma feasible? Cancer 2005;103(3):559–68.

[18] Morrissey DD, Andersen PE, Nesbit GM, et al. Endovascular management of hemorrhage in patients with head and neck cancer. Arch Otolaryngol Head Neck Surg 1997;123:15–9.

[19] Citardi MJ, Chaloupka JC, Son YH, et al. Management of carotid artery rupture by monitored endovascular therapeutic occlusion (1988–1994). Laryngoscope 1995;105:1086–92.

[20] Cohen J, Rad I. Contemporary management of carotid blowout. Curr Opin Otolaryngol Head Neck Surg 2004;12(2):110–5.

[21] Johnson MH. Carotid blow out syndromes. Endovascular Today 2003;15–8.

[22] Chaloupka JC, Roth TC, Putman CM, et al. Recurrent carotid blowout syndrome: diagnostic and therapeutic challenges in a newly recognized subgroup of patients. AJNR Am J Neuroradiol 1999; 20:1069–77.

[23] Chaloupka JC, Putman CM, Citardi MJ, et al. Endovascular therapy for the carotid blowout syndrome in head and neck surgical patients: diagnostic and managerial considerations. AJNR Am J Neuroradiol 1996;17:843–52.

[24] Ditmars ML, Klein SR, Bongard FS. Diagnosis and management of zone III carotid injuries. Injury 1997;28:515–20.

[25] Gaskill-Shipley MF, Tomsick TA. Angiography I: the evaluation of head and neck trauma. Neuroimaging Clin N Am 1996;6:607–24.

[26] Naidoo NM, Corr PD, Robbs JV, et al. Angiographic embolization in arterial trauma. Eur J Vasc Endovasc Surg 2000;19:77–81.

[27] Komiyama M, Nishikawa M, Kan M, et al. Endovascular treatment of intractable oronasal bleeding associated with severe craniofacial injury. J Trauma 1998;44:330–4.

[28] Gomez CR, May AK, Terry JB, et al. Endovascular therapy of traumatic injuries of the extracranial cerebral arteries. Crit Care Clin 1999;15: 789–809.

[29] Weiss VJ, Chaikof EL. Endovascular treatment of vascular injuries. Surg Clin North Am 1999;79: 653–65.

[30] Duke BJ, Ryu RK, Coldwell DM, et al. Treatment of blunt trauma to the carotid artery by using endovascular stents: an early experience. J Neurosurg 1997;87:825–9.

[31] Butterworth RJ, Thomas DJ, Wolfe JH, et al. Endovascular treatment of carotid dissecting aneurysms. Cerebrovasc Dis 1999;9:242–7.

[32] Higashida RT, Halbach VV, Tsai FY. Interventional neurovascular treatment of traumatic carotid and vertebral artery lesions: results in 234 cases. AJR Am J Roentgenol 1989;153:577–82.

[33] Huang A, Baker DM, al-Kutoubi A, et al. Endovascular stenting of internal artery false aneurysm. Eur J Vasc Endovasc Surg 1996;12:375–7.

[34] Hurst RW, Haskal ZJ, Zager E, et al. Endovascular stent treatment of cervical internal carotid artery aneurysms with parent vessel preservation. Surg Neurol 1998;50:313–7.

[35] Matsuura JH, Rosenthal D, Jerius H, et al. Traumatic carotid artery dissection and pseudoaneurysm treated with endovascular coils and stent. J Endovasc Surg 1997;4:339–43.

[36] Goodwin JR, Johnson MH. Carotid injury secondary to blunt head trauma: a case report. J Trauma 1994;37(1):119–22.

[37] Hemphill JC III, Gress DR, Halbach VV. Endovascular therapy of traumatic injuries of the intracranial cerebral arteries. Crit Care Clin 1999;15: 811–29.

[38] Kocer N, Kizilkilic O, Albayram S, et al. Treatment of iatrogenic internal carotid artery laceration and carotid cavernous fistula with endovascular stent-graft placement. AJNR Am J Neuroradiol 2002; 23(30):442–6.

[39] Sudhoff H, Stark T, Knorz S, et al. Massive epistaxis after rupture of intracavernous carotid artery aneurysm. Case report. Ann Otol Laryngol 2000;109: 776–8.

[40] Raymond J, Hardy J, Czepko R, et al. Arterial injuries in trans-sphenoidal surgery for pituitary adenoma: the role of angiography and endovascular treatment. AJNR Am J Neuroradiol 1997;18: 655–65.

[41] Teitelbaum GP, Halbach VV, Larsen DW, et al. Treatment of massive posterior epistaxis by detach-able coil embolization of a cavernous internal carotid artery aneurysm. Neuroradiology 1995;37:334–6.

[42] Chen D, Concus AP, Halbach VV, et al. Epistaxis originating from traumatic pseudoaneurysm of the internal carotid artery: diagnosis and endovascular therapy. Laryngoscope 1998;108:326–31.

[43] Koh E, Frazzini VI, Kagetsu NJ. Epistaxis: vascular anatomy, origins, and endovascular treatment. AJR Am J Roentgenol 2000;174:845–51.

[44] Guttmacher AE, Marchuk DA, White RI Jr. Hereditary hemorrhagic telangiectasia. N Engl J Med 1995;333:918–24.

[45] Fiorella ML, Ross D, Henderson KJ, White RI. Outcome of septal dermoplasty in patients with hereditary hemorrhagic telangiectasia. Laryngoscope 2005;115:301–5.

ELSEVIER
SAUNDERS

Neurosurg Clin N Am 16 (2005) 561–568

NEUROSURGERY
CLINICS
OF NORTH AMERICA

Percutaneous Spinal Interventions

Arun Paul Amar, MD[a],[*], Donald W. Larsen, MD[b],
George P. Teitelbaum, MD[b]

[a]Yale University School of Medicine, 333 Cedar Street, PO Box 208082,
New Haven, CT 06520–8082, USA
[b]Department of Neurological Surgery, Keck School of Medicine, University of Southern California
at Los Angeles, Los Angeles, CA 90033, USA

Interventional neuroradiology (INR) procedures of the spine are being performed with increasing frequency. These therapies complement and, in some cases, replace more conventional operations of the vertebral column and its contents. This article surveys the background, present application, and future horizons of several minimally invasive spinal interventions, including vertebroplasty and kyphoplasty, microcatheterization of the cervical epidural space via lumbar puncture for drug delivery, percutaneous intraspinal navigation, and percutaneous spinal fixation.

Percutaneous spinal osteoplasty

Percutaneous transpedicular polymethylmethacrylate (PMMA) vertebroplasty consists of the injection of acrylic cement into a partially collapsed vertebral body in an effort to relieve pain and augment mechanical stability in the management of vertebral compression fractures (VCFs) secondary to osteoporosis, aggressive hemangioma, myeloma, and osteolytic metastasis [1].

The mechanism underlying the palliative effects of vertebroplasty is not well elucidated. Injection of cement fortifies weakened segments of the vertebral column and may reduce pain by halting further compression, deformity, or micromotion. Alternatively, it has been proposed that the heat generated by the exothermic polymerization of PMMA damages pain-sensitive nerve endings within the vertebra and surrounding tissues. Others believe that analgesia results from leaching of the PMMA monomer, which may be toxic to nervous tissue. Thermal necrosis and toxic effects of the monomer may account for the antitumoral effects noted after vertebroplasty performed for spinal metastases [1].

A more recent variant, kyphoplasty, attempts to restore lost vertebral body height and reduce the kyphotic deformity associated with VCFs. In this method, an inflatable bone tamp (Kyphon, Santa Clara, California) is introduced percutaneously into the collapsed vertebral body. As the tamp is expanded, cancellous bone is compressed and the end plates are lifted, creating an *en masse* reduction. After tamp removal, the subsequent void can be filled with PMMA under lower pressure than that needed for conventional vertebroplasty, thus potentially reducing the risk of cement leakage [1].

The indications, technique, and outcomes of vertebroplasty and kyphoplasty have been widely published [1,2], but it is imperative to realize that neither procedure has ever been subjected to prospective randomized trials contrasting it to the natural history of VCFs. Furthermore, kyphoplasty and vertebroplasty have never been directly compared in any study. Thus, the purported benefits of one procedure over the other remain speculative.

Although percutaneous vertebroplasty under radiographic guidance was first performed in 1984, its use has grown exponentially in the past several years. The potential reasons for this phenomenon include the following:

* Corresponding author.
  E-mail address: amar@aya.yale.edu (A.P. Amar).

1. Aggressive marketing campaigns
2. Recent technical innovations and instrumentation enhancements (eg, kyphoplasty)
3. The enfranchisement of neurosurgeons, orthopedic surgeons, and other nonradiologist practitioners
4. The growing number of neurosurgeons with hybrid training in INR techniques
5. An ever-aging population with commensurate increases in the incidence of osteoporotic spinal compression fractures
6. The pervasive trend toward therapeutic minimalism

Patient selection

Osteoporotic compression fractures of the spine occur in 700,000 patients annually in the United States and are twice as frequent as fractures of the hip. Because of evolving demographic changes, the incidence of osteoporotic fractures is expected to increase fourfold during the next 50 years.

Eligible patients for vertebroplasty and kyphoplasty are those who suffer from disabling back pain or impaired mobility secondary to VCFs with varying pathologic findings. These procedures have been applied to all segments of the spine, including the sacrum [3].

Most patients have failed trials of conservative therapy, consisting of analgesics, bed rest, or external bracing. All patients should undergo various combinations of plain films, CT, radionuclide bone scans, or MRI to delineate the fracture pattern and to exclude other treatable causes of pain, such as a herniated intervertebral disk. Patients with severe spinal stenosis or intracanalicular fragments are excluded, although some centers in Europe have reported good results treating burst fractures of the thoracic and lumbar spine.

Because osteoporosis is a diffuse condition, patients may have multiple VCFs of uncertain age, because up to two thirds of osteoporotic compression fractures never come to clinical attention. In such instances, nuclear medicine imaging is useful to help differentiate the symptomatic level from incidentally discovered fractures. Increased activity revealed on bone scans is highly predictive of a positive clinical response to percutaneous spinal osteoplasty. In other patients, increased edema within the marrow space of the vertebral body on MRI, best visualized on sagittal T1-weighted spin echo sequences, is indicative of

a healing (acute or subacute) fracture amenable to these procedures. Up to three to four levels may be treated simultaneously at any one session [1].

History and physical examination also guide patient selection. Patients should be excluded if their pain fails to localize to the vicinity of the fracture, if the affected level is completely free of pain on palpation, or if there is an overwhelming radicular component to the pain, because the response to percutaneous spinal osteoplasty in such cases is unsatisfactory.

Surgical technique

The surgical technique of percutaneous spinal osteoplasty has been reviewed elsewhere [1,4]. Vertebroplasty is generally performed under local anesthesia along with intravenous neuroleptic anesthesia, using small doses of a narcotic for analgesia and a benzodiazepine for sedation and amnesia. Kyphoplasty, which is more painful because of the larger caliber of the instruments and the requirement for bone tamp inflation, is typically performed under general anesthesia.

Regardless of whether the procedure is conducted in the operating room or the INR suite, strict sterile protocol must be applied. After positioning the patient prone, the fractured level is visualized fluoroscopically and the needle entry sites overlying its pedicles are localized. For many cases of vertebroplasty, a unilateral approach is sufficient, but kyphoplasty requires placement of needles through both pedicles.

The skin and periosteum are locally anesthetized. A cannulated bone needle is inserted percutaneously and seated against the periosteum. Under fluoroscopic guidance, the needle is advanced through the middle portion of the pedicle into the anterior third of the collapsed vertebral body (Fig. 1). Recently, the adjunctive use of isocentric three-dimensional fluoroscopy-based navigation to guide placement of the cannula through the pedicle has been reported [5]. With image guidance, total duration and intraoperative fluoroscopy time were shorter than for procedures using biplanar fluoroscopy alone. Some groups advocate the use of CT during needle placement instead of fluoroscopic guidance.

Alternative techniques exist for gaining percutaneous access to the vertebral body, including the paraspinal route, which approaches the vertebral body from its posterolateral aspect. This trajectory is similar to that used for discography and arthroscopic disk excision. Proponents argue that

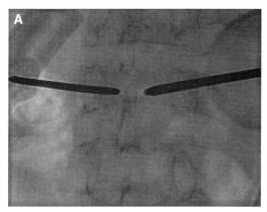
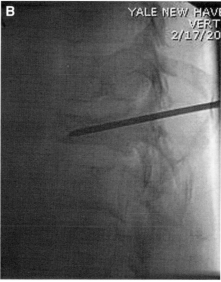

Fig. 1. Frontal (*A*) and lateral (*B*) radiographs demonstrate placement of cannulas through pedicles into the anterior third of the vertebral body.

the transpedicular approach places the nerve root and spinal cord at greater risk of injury, especially in the thoracic spine, where tolerances and pedicle sizes are smaller than in the lumbar region. Conversely, the paraspinal technique places several visceral structures at risk, including the lungs, kidneys, great vessels, segmental spinal arteries, and colon. Furthermore, with this approach, there may be a greater likelihood of cement leakage from the vertebral body once the cannula is removed [1].

Before cement delivery, some practitioners perform transosseous venography by injecting nonionic contrast material through the cannula. Rapid and brisk filling of the perimedullary veins or the inferior vena cava may indicate an increased risk of pulmonary embolism or epidural compression when cement is subsequently injected into the vertebral body. Venography may also help to evaluate the filling pattern and identify potential sites of PMMA leakage outside the vertebral body.

A variety of PMMA bone cements are commercially available, although many are not approved by the US Food and Drug Administration for spinal osteoplasty. The PMMA is mixed with an opacifying agent and, depending on operator preference, antibiotic powder. Under continuous fluoroscopic monitoring, cement is injected into the interstices of the vertebral body. Several delivery

systems are available, although we prefer a volumetrically controlled screw-system syringe for injection of the high-viscosity cement. Compared with conventional syringes, the threaded plunger affords greater control of the injection pressure and quantity of cement delivered.

During kyphoplasty, cement delivery is customarily achieved using a series of "bone filler device" (BFD) tubes. Each BFD must be manually loaded with cement, which is then injected into the kyphoplasty cavity by manually depressing an inner stylet. The high profile of the BFD cannulas and their stylets requires frequent repositioning of the image intensifier tube and table. Because each accommodates only a small volume, the BFDs must be exchanged frequently. This delivery method also places the operator's hands directly in the field of radiation. Because of these limitations, we substitute the screw-system syringe injector used to deliver cement during conventional vertebroplasty for the BFDs. This amalgam has several merits over the customary means of cement delivery during kyphoplasty [6].

Care must be taken to avoid extrusion of cement beyond the confines of the vertebral body and inadvertent filling of the spinal canal, neural foramina, intervertebral disk spaces, or vertebral venous plexus. Cement is introduced until at least 70% of the vertebral body is filled. Ideally, the cement permeates the anterior three

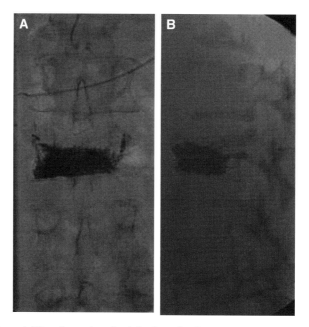

Fig. 2. Frontal (*A*) and lateral (*B*) radiographs after injection of polymethylmethacrylate cement mixed with barium. Ideally, the cement permeates the anterior three quarters of the vertebral body and at least two thirds of its transverse dimension.

quarters of the vertebral body and at least two thirds of its transverse dimension (Fig. 2). At the conclusion of the procedure, the needle is withdrawn. Antibiotic ointment and a sterile dressing are placed over the skin puncture site. The patient is placed on bed rest for 2 hours while the cement cures into a hardened state and is then discharged to home the same day unless general anesthesia is used.

Results

The response to vertebroplasty and kyphoplasty is generally favorable, with most series demonstrating a 75% to 90% likelihood of significant pain relief in properly selected patients [1,2]. Narcotic and analgesic requirements typically decrease. Sleep, ambulation, and other activities of daily living are improved. In many cases, pain relief occurs immediately. Results are durable, although recurrence of pain may occur from the development of a new VCF at an additional level.

When kyphoplasty was introduced, one of the earliest claims advanced by its proponents was the potential to restore lost vertebral body height and reduce the associated kyphosis. Some studies lend credence to this contention. Quantitative morphometric analysis before and after kyphoplasty demonstrates a significant reduction in vertebral body deformity as result of treatment [7]. In contrast, other studies have failed to demonstrate any restoration of vertebral body height [8]. Nevertheless, patients in the latter studies experienced profound clinical improvement. Thus, the impact of kyphoplasty on spinal alignment and the relation of this effect to pain relief remain unresolved controversies.

Complications of vertebroplasty and kyphoplasty include pulmonary embolism of cement, which can be fatal. Extrusion of PMMA cement beyond the confines of the vertebral body is observed commonly (up to 73% in some series). Although most cases are asymptomatic, several instances of spinal cord compression and myelopathy have been reported, with only modest recovery in neurologic function after emergency laminectomy. Nerve root compression with radicular pain or weakness may result from cement extrusion into the neural foramen. Other potential risks include cerebrospinal fluid (CSF) leak and infection, which may require corpectomy. Because most patients undergoing these procedures are elderly, pneumonia, myocardial infarction, and other medical complications may also occur [1].

Future directions

PMMA cement has a number of undesirable attributes, including the potential for thermal necrosis and its inability to integrate with the skeleton. In addition to acrylic polymers, such as PMMA, the transpedicular vertebroplasty technique permits the percutaneous delivery of several biocompatible materials into the vertebral body. Future treatment of compression fractures is likely to consist of injecting materials like hydroxyapatite, hormones, osteogenic growth factors, allograft or autograft, and other agents that induce bone regeneration. Biodegradable bone mineral substitutes that resorb as the bone remodels are currently being evaluated, as are osteoconductive materials, such as coral exoskeleton [1]. Newer systems for vertebral augmentation are likely to combine minimally invasive surgical access with bioactive injectable material to restore vertebral body height and sagittal alignment, provide structural stability by sustaining physiologic loads, and allow for the incorporation of graft material into native vertebral bone [1,9].

Cervical epidural microcatheterization

Deposition of anti-inflammatory or analgesic medication into the epidural space is a useful adjunct in the management of several spinal disorders, including pain of discogenic and spondylitic origin [10]. In addition to providing temporary relief of pain, the response to epidural drug therapy may help to predict surgical outcomes, thus maximizing the likelihood of a successful operation. Because these degenerative changes can affect every vertebral level, epidural analgesia and steroid infusion over long segments are potentially beneficial. The effect of this therapy is restricted to the spinal levels adjacent to the site of delivery, however, because of limited diffusion of medication within the epidural space. In practice, epidural injections are most commonly performed in the lumbar region, because anatomic factors make thoracic and cervical epidural access more hazardous. Risks of direct puncture of the latter areas include spinal cord injury and myelopathy, infection, bleeding, and pain.

Contemporary microcatheter technology has allowed remote access of confined anatomic spaces within the vascular system. The flexibility and low profile of these new devices minimize trauma and distortion of nearby structures. Application of endovascular technology and techniques allow placement of a microcatheter into the cervical epidural space via lumbar puncture for the purpose of drug delivery.

Surgical technique

The patient is brought to the INR suite and positioned prone. The midline of the lower back is prepared and draped sterilely. Under fluoroscopy, one of the lumbar interspinous spaces is selected for access. Local anesthesia is injected into the subcutaneous tissue overlying this interspace. An 18-gauge Tuohy needle is then introduced between the spinous processes and directed under fluoroscopic guidance to the spinolaminar line. The stylet is withdrawn, and the needle is gradually advanced while attempting to inject small aliquots of air through a 10-mL syringe until the epidural space is encountered. Correct needle placement is confirmed by the injection of radiographic contrast [10].

Next, a 2.3-French angiography microcatheter with a coaxial 0.018-inch steerable guidewire is introduced through the lumen of the Tuohy needle. Under biplane fluoroscopic imaging, the guidewire is advanced cephalad through the epidural space, followed by the trailing microcatheter. Patients frequently report a pressure-like discomfort during transit through the thoracic region. Once the cervical epidural space is reached, the guidewire is removed and a small amount of additional contrast is injected to confirm the absence of intravascular or intrathecal filling. Steroid medication can then be delivered through the microcatheter. Narcotics are avoided at this region because of the risk of respiratory depression. As with other epidural or nerve root blocks, reproduction of the patient's symptoms during the injection often signifies the appropriate anatomic level. In patients with concurrent spondylitic and discogenic changes of the thoracic spine, the catheter can be withdrawn to the symptomatic site, where additional steroid and narcotics are administered for regional analgesia.

Results

More than 40 cervical epidural microcatheterization procedures have been performed. Eligible patients suffered from spondylitic or discogenic disease of the cervical spine and presented with arm, neck, shoulder, or interscapular pain. In addition, several had radicular or local pain referable to degenerative changes in the thoracic spine.

In follow-up averaging 12 weeks (range: 4–12 weeks), all patients reported relief of varying extent and duration [10]. The results of cervical epidural steroid administration via this technique were similar to those with lumbar epidural steroid treatment and are generally consistent with the variable efficacy of epidural corticosteroids reported in the literature.

No procedures were aborted because of anatomic constraints or technical limitations, even among patients with severe spinal stenosis. There has been no clinically apparent infection, epidural hematoma, arachnoiditis, spinal cord injury, nerve root damage, CSF leak, or other complication.

Percutaneous intraspinal navigation

Recent advances in catheter technology and imaging allow potential new applications outside the vascular system. A percutaneous approach to cerebral access using the spinal subarachnoid space has been devised and tested in cadavers [11]. In this method, needle puncture allows for placement of an arterial introduction sheath within the lumbar cistern. Guidewires and catheters can then be introduced through this sheath and traverse the subarachnoid space until the intracranial contents are encountered. Intraspinal navigation and monitoring of guidewire and/or catheter position may be conducted with standard fluoroscopy. Alternatively, steady-state free precession MRI guidance may be used to track device position [12]. This imaging modality provides adequate contrast and temporal resolution to facilitate real-time MRI-guided intracranial and intraspinal navigation.

The subarachnoid space ventral and dorsal to the spinal cord has been traversed with relative ease. In limited analysis of cadaveric specimens, neither the guidewire nor the catheter has caused spinal cord violation or laceration [11]. No significant disruption of the epidural vasculature was identified.

In theory, percutaneous intraspinal navigation may serve many potential functions. Intracranial applications could possibly include ventricular catheterization, brain biopsy, depth electrode implantation, electrophysiologic recording, delivery of interstitial brachytherapy, and thermal ablation [11]. Endospinal MRI of the thoracic and cervical cord may be performed by using an antenna and/or guidewire introduced into the subarachnoid space via percutaneous intraspinal navigation techniques. When compared with images obtained from a linear surface coil, images obtained with the endospinal coil showed significant signal-to-noise ratio (SNR) gains [13]. This advantage may allow superior imaging in spinal cord injury and other disease states. The high SNR of the endospinal coil might also be exploited for magnetic resonance spectroscopy and diffusion-weighed imaging of the spinal cord, which have not been optimized using current surface coil technology [13].

Although percutaneous intraspinal navigation has only been studied in cadaver and canine experiments to date, continued evolution of catheter and imaging technology may allow its clinical application in the future.

Percutaneous spinal fixation

Back and neck pain affects up to 80% of Americans at some time in their lives. Greater than 150,000 lumbar and nearly 200,000 cervical spinal fusions are performed each year to treat common spinal disorders, such as degenerative disk disease, spondylolisthesis, and vertebral column trauma.

Posterior instrumentation is frequently used to augment anterior and posterior lumbar interbody fusions as well as cervical and thoracic fixation. Pedicle screws and rods are commonly used for this purpose. Traditional open surgical methods for the insertion of posterior instrumentation have several disadvantages, including the risk of significant blood loss, the potential for serious infections, and the need for extensive paraspinous muscular dissection to expose the anatomic landmarks for screw insertion, achieve proper screw trajectory, and develop a suitable fusion bed [14]. The tissue injury resulting from this dissection may lead to muscular denervation and necrosis, resulting in prolonged postoperative pain and disability.

Because of these limitations, tissue-sparing techniques to achieve spinal fixation have been sought. Minimally invasive approaches have been applied to a wide range of procedures, including anterior, posterior, and transforaminal lumbar interbody fusions; posterolateral onlay fusion; and pedicle screw and rod placement [14].

Early in the evolution of minimally invasive spinal fixation, endoscopes were used to minimize the size of the incision required to develop the surgical corridor. In contrast, the Sextant system (Medronic, Minneapolis, Minnesota) enables the minimally invasive placement of percutaneous pedicle screws and rods in a subfascial anatomic position similar to that of traditional open techniques using fluoroscopic guidance [14–16]. The Sextant system consists of specially designed, cannulated pedicle screws connected via a precontoured rod. A disadvantage of the precurved rod is difficulty in passing it between three adjacent pedicle screws or in the presence of bony impediments to rigid rod placement.

Recently, a new percutaneous minimally invasive spinal fixation system based on pedicle screws and inflatable rods was described [17]. The rods are inserted in a flexible state and harden after deployment, thus enabling them to be able to traverse and conform to complex pathways between multiple screws (Fig. 3). The rods are filled with a novel expandable composite of epoxy polymer and graphite fiber matrix, which exhibits strength comparable to that of metallic rods. All system components were found to be biocompatible and nonferromagnetic and to produce little magnetic resonance artifact. Compression and torque results for the construct were found to be comparable to those of standard metallic pedicle screw and rod fixation systems. The new system displayed a superior modulus of elasticity relative to standard surgical devices, however. The new system endured 5 million cycles of repetitive compressions without breakage or significant wear. The epoxy polymer used to inflate the

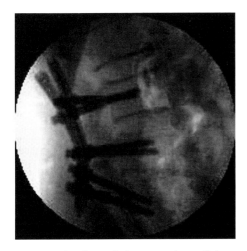

Fig. 3. Lateral radiograph demonstrating pedicle screw and inflatable rod spinal fixation system inserted percutaneously.

flexible rods cured to approximately 53% of its final strength in 90 minutes, with a maximum external rod temperature of 40.5°C and no thermal damage to paraspinous musculature and other adjacent tissues in animal studies.

Because of its minimally invasive insertion, the new pedicle screw and rod fixation system may potentially reduce procedural morbidity, decrease paraspinous muscle denervation and necrosis, and speed postoperative recovery. Device characteristics eliminate the need for rod shaping and facilitate rod placement between more than two pedicle screws. These results support the concept that composite devices can be constructed in situ within the body using minimally invasive percutaneous INR techniques.

References

[1] Amar AP, Larsen DW, Esnaashari N, et al. Percutaneous transpedicular polymethylmethacrylate vertebroplasty for the treatment of spinal compression fractures. Neurosurgery 2001;49(5):1105–15.

[2] Burton AW, Rhines LD, Mendel E. Vertebroplasty and kyphoplasty: a comprehensive review. Neurosurg Focus 2005;18(3):E1–9.

[3] Deen HG, Nottmeier EW. Balloon kyphoplasty for treatment of sacral insufficiency fractures. Neurosurg Focus 2005;18(3):E1–5.

[4] Wong W, Mathis JM. Vertebroplasty and kyphoplasty: techniques for avoiding complications and pitfalls. Neurosurg Focus 2005;18(3):E1–10.

[5] Villavicencio AT, Burneikiene S, Bulsara KR, et al. Intraoperative three-dimensional fluoro-based CT guidance for percutaneous kyphoplasty. Neurosurg Focus 2005;18(3):E1–7.

[6] Amar AP, Larsen DW, Teitelbaum GP. Use of a screw-syringe injector for cement delivery during kyphoplasty: technical report. Neurosurgery 2003;53(2):380–3.

[7] Ledlie JT, Renfro MB. Kyphoplasty decreases the number and severity of morphometrically defined vertebral deformities. Neurosurg Focus 2005;18(3):E1–5.

[8] Feltes C, Fountas KN, Machinis T, et al. Immediate and early post-operative pain relief after kyphoplasty without significant restoration of vertebral body height in acute osteoporotic vertebral body fractures. Neurosurg Focus 2005;18(3):E1–4.

[9] Lam S, Khoo LT. A novel percutaneous system for bone graft delivery and containment for elevation and stabilization of vertebral compression fractures. Technical note. Neurosurg Focus 2005;18(3):E1–7.

[10] Amar AP, Wang MY, Larsen DW, et al. Microcatheterization of the cervical epidural space via

lumbar puncture: technical note. Neurosurgery 2001;48(5):1183–7.

[11] Purdy PD, Replogle RE, Pride GL, et al. Percutaneous intraspinal navigation: feasibility study of a new and minimally invasive approach to the spinal cord and brain in cadavers. AJNR Am J Neuroradiol 2003;24:361–5.

[12] Rappard G, Metzger GJ, Fleckenstein JL, et al. MR-guided catheter navigation of the intracranial subarachnoid space. AJNR Am J Neuroradiol 2003; 24:626–9.

[13] Rappard G, Metzger GJ, Weatherall PT, et al. Interventional MR imaging with an endospinal imaging coil: preliminary results with anatomic imaging of the canine and cadaver spinal cord. AJNR Am J Neuroradiol 2004;25:835–9.

[14] Foley KT, Holly LT, Schwender JD. Minimally invasive lumbar fusion. Spine 2003;28(15 Suppl): S26–35.

[15] Foley KT, Gupta S. Percutaneous pedicle screw fixation of the lumbar spine: preliminary clinical results. J Neurosurg Spine 2002;97(1):7–12.

[16] Khoo LT, Palmer S, Laich DT, et al. Minimally invasive percutaneous posterior lumbar interbody fusion. Neurosurgery 2002;51(5 Suppl):S166–81.

[17] Teitelbaum GP, Shaolian S, McDougall CG, et al. New percutaneously inserted spinal fixation system. Spine 2004;29(6):703–9.

ELSEVIER
SAUNDERS

Neurosurg Clin N Am 16 (2005) 569–574

NEUROSURGERY
CLINICS
OF NORTH AMERICA

Index

Note: Page numbers of article titles are in **bold face** type.

Changing Your Address?

Make sure your subscription changes too! When you notify us of your new address, you can help make our job easier by including an exact copy of your Clinics label number with your old address (see illustration below.) This number identifies you to our computer system and will speed the processing of your address change. Please be sure this label number accompanies your old address and your corrected address—you can send an old Clinics label with your number on it or just copy it exactly and send it to the address listed below.

We appreciate your help in our attempt to give you continuous coverage. Thank you.

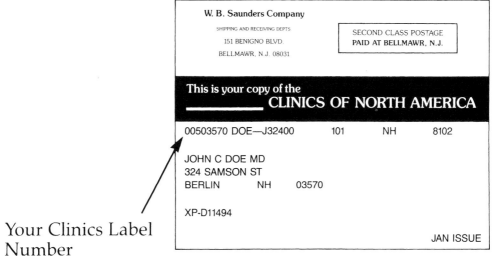

Your Clinics Label Number
Copy it exactly or send your label along with your address to:
W.B. Saunders Company, Customer Service
Orlando, FL 32887-4800
Call Toll Free 1-800-654-2452

Please allow four to six weeks for delivery of new subscriptions and for processing address changes.

Practice, Current, Hardbound:
SATISFACTION GUARANTEED

YES! Please start my subscription to the **CLINICS** checked below with the ❑ first issue of the calendar year or ❑ current issues. If not completely satisfied with my first issue, I may write "cancel" on the invoice and return it within 30 days at no further obligation.

Please Print:

Name _____

Address_____

City_____ State _____ ZIP _____

Method of Payment

❑ Check (payable to **Elsevier**; add the applicable sales tax for your area)

❑ VISA   ❑ MasterCard   ❑ AmEx   ❑ Bill me

Card number _____ Exp. date _____

Signature _____

Staple this to your purchase order to expedite delivery

❑ **Adolescent Medicine Clinics**
- ❑ Individual $95
- ❑ Institutions $133
- ❑ *In-training $48

❑ **Anesthesiology**
- ❑ Individual $175
- ❑ Institutions $270
- ❑ *In-training $88

❑ **Cardiology**
- ❑ Individual $170
- ❑ Institutions $266
- ❑ *In-training $85

❑ **Chest Medicine**
- ❑ Individual $185
- ❑ Institutions $285

❑ **Child and Adolescent Psychiatry**
- ❑ Individual $175
- ❑ Institutions $265
- ❑ *In-training $88

❑ **Critical Care**
- ❑ Individual $165
- ❑ Institutions $266
- ❑ *In-training $83

❑ **Dental**
- ❑ Individual $150
- ❑ Institutions $242

❑ **Emergency Medicine**
- ❑ Individual $170
- ❑ Institutions $263
- ❑ *In-training $85
  - ❑ Send CME info

❑ **Facial Plastic Surgery**
- ❑ Individual $199
- ❑ Institutions $300

❑ **Foot and Ankle**
- Individual $160
- Institutions $232

❑ **Gastroenterology**
- ❑ Individual $190
- ❑ Institutions $276

❑ **Gastrointestinal Endoscopy**
- ❑ Individual $190
- ❑ Institutions $276

❑ **Hand**
- ❑ Individual $205
- ❑ Institutions $319

❑ **Heart Failure (NEW in 2005!)**
- ❑ Individual $99
- ❑ Institutions $149
- ❑ *In-training $49

❑ **Hematology/ Oncology**
- ❑ Individual $210
- ❑ Institutions $315

❑ **Immunology & Allergy**
- ❑ Individual $165
- ❑ Institutions $266

❑ **Infectious Disease**
- ❑ Individual $165
- ❑ Institutions $272

❑ **Clinics in Liver Disease**
- ❑ Individual $165
- ❑ Institutions $234

❑ **Medical**
- ❑ Individual $140
- ❑ Institutions $244
- ❑ *In-training $70
  - ❑ Send CME info

❑ **MRI**
- ❑ Individual $190
- ❑ Institutions $290
- ❑ *In-training $95
  - ❑ Send CME info

❑ **Neuroimaging**
- ❑ Individual $190
- ❑ Institutions $290
- ❑ *In-training $95
  - ❑ Send CME inf0

❑ **Neurologic**
- ❑ Individual $175
- ❑ Institutions $275

❑ **Obstetrics & Gynecology**
- ❑ Individual $175
- ❑ Institutions $288

❑ **Occupational and Environmental Medicine**
- ❑ Individual $120
- ❑ Institutions $166
- ❑ *In-training $60

❑ **Ophthalmology**
- ❑ Individual $190
- ❑ Institutions $325

❑ **Oral & Maxillofacial Surgery**
- ❑ Individual $180
- ❑ Institutions $280
- ❑ *In-training $90

❑ **Orthopedic**
- ❑ Individual $180
- ❑ Institutions $295
- ❑ *In-training $90

❑ **Otolaryngologic**
- ❑ Individual $199
- ❑ Institutions $350

❑ **Pediatric**
- ❑ Individual $135
- ❑ Institutions $246
- ❑ *In-training $68
  - ❑ Send CME info

❑ **Perinatology**
- ❑ Individual $155
- ❑ Institutions $237
- ❑ *In-training $78
  - ❑ Send CME inf0

❑ **Plastic Surgery**
- ❑ Individual $245
- ❑ Institutions $370

❑ **Podiatric Medicine & Surgery**
- ❑ Individual $170
- ❑ Institutions $266

❑ **Primary Care**
- ❑ Individual $135
- ❑ Institutions $223

❑ **Psychiatric**
- ❑ Individual $170
- ❑ Institutions $288

❑ **Radiologic**
- ❑ Individual $220
- ❑ Institutions $331
- ❑ *In-training $110
  - ❑ Send CME info

❑ **Sports Medicine**
- ❑ Individual $180
- ❑ Institutions $277

❑ **Surgical**
- ❑ Individual $190
- ❑ Institutions $299
- ❑ *In-training $95

❑ **Thoracic Surgery (formerly Chest Surgery)**
- ❑ Individual $175
- ❑ Institutions $255
- ❑ *In-training $88

❑ **Urologic**
- ❑ Individual $195
- ❑ Institutions $307
- ❑ *In-training $98
  - ❑ Send CME info

*To receive in-training rate, orders must be accompanied by the name of affiliated institution, dates of residency and signature of coordinator on institution letterhead. Orders will be billed at the individual rate until proof of resident status is received.

Order your subscription today. Simply complete and detach this card and drop it in the mail to receive the best clinical information in your field.

BUSINESS REPLY MAIL

FIRST-CLASS MAIL   PERMIT NO 7135   ORLANDO FL

POSTAGE WILL BE PAID BY ADDRESSEE

PERIODICALS ORDER FULFILLMENT DEPT
ELSEVIER
6277 SEA HARBOR DR
ORLANDO FL 32821-9816